Older Adult-Led
Health Promotion in
Urban Communities

Older Adult-Led
Health Promotion in
Urban Communities

Models and Interventions

Melvin Delgado

ROWMAN & LITTLEFIELD PUBLISHERS, INC.
Lanham • Boulder • New York • Toronto • Plymouth, UK

ROWMAN & LITTLEFIELD PUBLISHERS, INC.

Published in the United States of America
by Rowman & Littlefield Publishers, Inc.
A wholly owned subsidary of The Rowman & Littlefield Publishing Group, Inc.
4501 Forbes Boulevard, Suite 200, Lanham, Maryland 20706
www.rowmanlittlefield.com

Estover Road
Plymouth PL6 7PY
United Kingdom

British Library Cataloguing in Publication Information Available

Library of Congress Cataloging-in-Publication Data

Delgado, Melvin.
   Older adult-led health promotion in urban communities : models and
interventions / Melvin Delgado.
       p. ; cm.
   Includes bibliographical references and indexes.
   ISBN-13: 978-0-7425-6335-3 (cloth : alk. paper)
   ISBN-10: 0-7425-6335-9 (cloth : alk. paper)
   ISBN 13: 978-0-7425-6887-7 (electronic)
   ISBN 10: 0-7425-6887-3 (electronic)
   1. Health promotion—United States. 2. Older people—United States.
   3. Minorities—United States. 4. Urban health—United States. I. Title.
   [DNLM: 1. Health Promotion—methods—United States. 2. Aged—United
States. 3. Minority Health—United States. 4. Urban Health—United States.
WA 590 D352o 2009]
RA427.8.D45 2009
362.10973—dc22   2008025943

Printed in the United States of America

⊗™ The paper used in this publication meets the minimum requirements of
American National Standard for Information Sciences—Permanence of Paper
for Printed Library Materials, ANSI/NISO Z39.48-1992.

This book is dedicated to Denise, Laura, and Barbara.

Contents

List of Figures and Tables

Acknowledgments

I wish to thank Dorothy "Jody" Miesel and David Sadownick, research assistants, for their work on this book, and my Boston University School of Social Work Gerontology colleagues (Scott Geron, Judith Gonyea, and Robert Hudson) for their inspiring work in the field of aging, and Beth Eldridge of Older Women's Network, New South Wales, Australia, for her assistance in providing a wealth of information on this program.

SECTION 1:
SETTING THE CONTEXT

"The United States is in the midst of a profound demographic change: The rapid aging of its population. . . . The effects of this older age profile will reverberate throughout the American economy and society in the next 50 years. Preparing for these changes involves more than the study of demographic trends; it also requires an understanding of the growing diversity within the older population."

(Himes, 2002, p. 3)

1

~~

Overview

"As we all learned in grade school, America, specifically Florida, was 'discovered' by explorers searching for the fountain of youth. . . . Five hundred or so years later, many of us are still not willing to give up the quest. If anything, we seem to be even more determined in our pursuit of the secrets leading to perpetual youth. What spurs on this quest is the fact that we can all see that some people do, in fact, age better than others."

(Budrys, 2003, p. 1)

The quest for health in this society is often equated with youthfulness, as noted in Budrys' quote at the top of this chapter. It is rare that a day goes by in this country when the subject of health does not receive national attention in the public media. Invariably, this attention focuses on diseases and illnesses, the costs of providing health care, and how to finance it in the present and not-too-distant future. Garrett and Martini (2007) comment that an aging population does result in increased costs as the result of certain chronic diseases.

Chronic diseases, for example, account for 75 percent of health care costs per year ("Healthy Messages," 2003). However, an aging population also results in decreases in health care costs in pregnancy and infertility, substance abuse, and mental health conditions, for example. How best to prevent or mitigate the consequences of ill health, however, is generally overlooked (Budrys, 2003). Consequently, the subject of health in the public's eye is invariably one that is fraught with negative images and

3

fears. When positive images come to mind, they usually do not refer to older adults!

Not unexpectedly, when health is addressed in some form, older adults tend to be viewed as an age group not benefiting from prevention or health promotion (Fried, 2000; Nolan, 2001; Richard et al., 2004; K. Miller & Dabson, 2005). This is particularly the case involving low-income and low-wealth older adults of color, for example, who rarely are the subject of news headlines involving the graying of the country. These age and ethnic/racial-group oversights, if you wish, are quite pervasive and symbolic of how a nation that "worships" youth actually thinks of its senior citizens. When ageism is combined with racism and classism, the outcomes can be quite devastating for older adults of color who, in essence, occupy an invisible position within this landscape (R. Clark, 2004).

Health promotion as a national and international field has grown considerably over the past two decades, with a number of exciting new developments being reported in the professional literature and in professional conferences of various types, such as youth-led health promotion (Delgado & Zhou, 2008). Cattan (2001), in a review of the field, nevertheless concludes what numerous experts have noted: that the field of health promotion for older adults has suffered from a lack of strategic planning and investment of appropriate resources. In other words, there is "a lack of imagination" when it comes to older adult health promotion. Marshall and Altpeter (2005), for example, in commenting on social work as a profession and older adult health promotion, stress the need for the profession to play a more active and leadership role in this field.

Historically, health promotion has generally been considered the exclusive domain of children, youth, and adults, but not older adults, as evidenced by the abundance of books on the subject. It is not unusual that the typical image of older adults held by the general public is that of a person who is frail (R. W. Johnson & Wiener, 2006). Further, it is also one of a person who cannot contribute much to their family, community, and society. In essence, someone who is at best occupying space! However, just as health promotion is not the exclusive domain of any one group, neither is it restricted to any particular health status (Minkler, Schauffler, & Clements-Nolle, 1999). Health promotion is for all age groups, regardless of their age and health status. Meecham (2006), Duggleby and Raudonis(2006), Lafreniere (2004), J. Richardson (2002), and Buckley (2002), among others, advance the proposition that health promotion also has a prominent place in palliative care, a population group that has almost universally been overlooked by the field, for example. Thus, there is no stage in the life cycle that cannot benefit from health promotion.

Ageism may also have played a role because of thinking premised on the adage "you cannot teach an old dog new tricks," reflecting professional bias about how arduous it is to introduce new ways of thinking among older adults. (Arean, 2003). This bias against older adults is, at least in part, the result of a belief that older adults have lived a long life and there is little need or benefit to changing behavior that can compromise their health (Wilken, 2002). Society, as a result, is best to invest resources on population groups that both have a future but are also in a position to continue to contribute to the gross national product!

Bias against older adults in our society gets manifested in a variety of direct and indirect ways. M. M. Lee, Carpenter, and Meyers (2006), in a study of representations of older adults in television advertisements, found that older adults were generally relegated to non-youth-oriented networks and to daytime hours. Further, the roles they played on television could be considered incidental to promote a "circumscribed, stereotyped set of products and services." Vickers (2007), in turn, traces the influence of the media over the past thirty years on popular views of older adults by the general population and older adult views of themselves, and raises concerns as well as hopes for the future regarding media images of older adults in our society.

The health care field, unfortunately, is not exempt from engaging in this form of bias and systematic discrimination (Vann, 2006). Gruman (2004, p. 3) makes a similar observation of this bias: "But health promotion directed to older adults is not getting a lot of traction, even as baby boomers are starting to deal with their aging parents' medical, money and mobility concerns . . . why are the prospects for health promotion for older Americans so dim on the policy radar screen? Again, the Three A's —ageism, affordability and accommodation." Freedman (1999, p. 16), in turn, notes: "The problem with so much wringing about the aging in America is not only that it distorts the purported crisis but also that it is blinding us to the benefits of an aging society. . . . Graying is about more than just paying, and the aging of America is about more than entitlements and the cost of supporting a much larger older population."

This disempowering and limiting perspective of older adults identified by Gruman (2004), Freedman (1999), and others effectively hampers the health field, and health promotion initiatives in particular, from developing exciting innovative approaches for reaching this population group. Further, and probably more significantly, it effectively eliminates the consideration of older adults playing key decision-making roles in how older adult health promotion gets conceptualized and implemented. In effect, it sells the field and older adults short. It essentially becomes a conceptual stretch to offer health promotion targeting older adults, and an even greater stretch to envision older adults actually leading these efforts. There is a well-grounded understanding of what actions older adults need to take in order to live longer and healthier lives. However, the lack of comprehensive older adult health promotion has acted as a significant barrier to doing so (Center for the Advancement of Health, 2006).

A quick review of published books written on health promotion, which are too numerous to list here, will uncover only four books specifically devoted to older adult health promotion (Chivas & Stears, 2001; Haber, 2007; Keller & Fleury, 1999; P. O'Neill, 2002). The first book looks at health promotion from a British perspective, and the latter three books focus on the United States. With notable exceptions, older adults are not considered a population group worthy of attention, and based upon the large gap in years since these books were published, not much has gone on in this field related to older adults to warrant several books on the subject. However, this is not true based upon an extensive review of published scholarly articles, and of practices in the field that have not been reported in the literature (Mitchell, Wiener, & Gage, 2006). None of these books specially addresses older adults of color, which is probably the most at-risk subgroup of an ever-increasing older adult population within the United States.

Nestle and Cowell (1990) were one of the earliest health promoters to identify low-income groups of color as being a high priority for the field, even though reaching this population group would prove challenging, in this case for nutrition education but also for other areas. Young (1993), three years later, focused specifically on older adults of color and advanced disease-specific health promotion strategies that emphasized communication strategies as a model for older adults-of-color health promotion. Yee and Weaver (1994) also identified the potential of health promotion for helping older adults of color. However, the progress these and other scholars advocated almost two decades ago has yet to be fully realized.

The National Hispanic Council on Aging (2005) identifies health promotion, disease prevention, education, and outreach as primary areas of significance. They recommended initiatives that systematically engage and build upon community-based organizations as a strategy for minimizing institutional barriers to health care for Latino older adults. There is recognition that older adults are part of the basic fabric of Latino communities, and as a result, every effort must be made to reach this group through the social and religious institutions they belong to. These institutions speak their language, understand their culture, and most important, are trusted. As a result, there is little controversy within the Latino community concerning the importance of community-based coalitions of lay helpers (*promotoras*) and organizations to facilitate service delivery to Latino older adults and prevent, control, and manage diabetes and associated disorders. Promotoras, for example, have been found to be effective in allowing Latinos to make their homes safer from pesticides (Foster-Cox et al., 2007).

Community health forums have been highly recommended as a way of facilitating the bridge between formal and informal service providers (Jennings-Sanders, 2003). Small group discussions called *"Ollas del Buen Comer"* (Skillets for Healthy Eating), making diet and exercise an important part of daily living, have been found to be an effective method of reaching Latino older adults, particularly when these forums systematically include and build upon community institutions (Sotomayor, Pawlik, & Dominguez, 2007). The case study of the Older Women's Network presented in chapter 10 utilizes small group discussions as a means of addressing older women's health needs and concerns, as well as emphasizing wellness strategies.

Hosay (2003) stresses the importance of the unique roles and contributions health care providers can play in health promotion and health education efforts for older adults. Greater recognition of health promotion efforts targeting older adults is needed to overcome bias and lower expectations of how older adults can increase their knowledge of health and health-promoting behaviors. Morley and Flaherty (2002), in turn, note that health promotion can range from simple but effective interventions—such as an influenza vaccination that transpires in an office—to complex interventions that transpire in community-based settings. This flexibility in approach toward health promotion and older adults lends itself to a wide range of local circumstances and local goals influencing the nature and extent of interventions.

Recently, the U.S. Administration on Aging (2006) announced an initiative (the Evidence-Based Disease Prevention Program) that highlights the importance of prevention for older adults, and this bodes well for the field of health promotion. Nakasato and Carnes (2006) advance the concept of "successful aging" as a means of capturing a wide range of interventions, including health promotion, that can be implemented with older adults as a specific target, and provide a more "positive" view of the aging process and potential contributions of older adults. The absence of a positive or affirming view on aging essentially reflects a serious bias in this country that effectively equates aging with disease and death. This perspective must be avoided at all cost by the field of health promotion.

How health is defined by older adults themselves, addressed in greater detail in chapter 5, becomes an integral part of how health promotion gets conceptualized and carried out in day-to-day practice. De La Rue and Coulson (2003), for example, specifically look at how health and well-being are defined for older rural women, and raise important implications for how perceptions of health influence help-seeking patterns and the delivery of health care. Promoting physical and mental health can be considered as important as preventing diseases (Missouri Rural Health Association 2006). Penprase (2006) stresses the importance of actively and meaningfully including older adults in any comprehensive planning for health services. This participation helps ensure that services reflect the perceptions and expectations of the ultimate beneficiaries of these services.

Klinedinst (2005), in turn, advances a program targeting low-income urban older adults and nutrition education, and the need for programming to be contextualized to take into account the reality facing these consumers. These and other efforts addressed in this book represent but a small percentage of the health promotion activities that can be found throughout the country that have focused on older adults and take into account how context influences the planning, implementation, and research of health promotion initiatives. Consequently, the field of older adult health promotion is vibrant and expanding in a manner usually associated with any field full of promise and potential. Older adult-led health promotion represents the latest and, arguably, the most exciting stage in this evolution.

This assessment of the field of health promotion and older adults takes on even greater significance in light of how much the United States' older adult population has increased over the past decade, and the demographic projections for this group in the next twenty-five years, as covered in chapter 2. Health promotion, as argued by this book, is not the exclusive domain of the young. Further, there is no reason why older adults cannot play leadership roles in designing and implementing health promotion projects. For health promotion to achieve maximum potential in society, it must embrace all age groups and subgroups, since no group, regardless of social characteristics, must be considered a vital part of society (Nakasato & Carnes, 2006). Ignoring a significant age group such as older adults effectively limits society's abilities to maximize the potential contribution of all of its members (Davis & Chesbro, 2003; National Association of Area Agencies on Aging, 2007). Older adults, in essence, represent an important social capital for this and all other societies and are worthy of investment in their well-being (Hawe & Shiell, 2000; Newman & Goff, 2006; Sander & Putnam, 2006).

This book is specifically devoted to older adults, as noted in the title. However, whenever possible, based upon available information, particular attention will be paid to urban older adults of color who are of low income and low wealth, a subpopulation group that is growing demographically and presents a series of challenges for both providers across disciplines and academics/researchers. This group is singled out because of a host of socioeconomic-political factors that have them entering into older adulthood in much poorer health when compared with their white, non-Latino counterparts (Angel & Whitfield, 2007; Dancy & Ralston, 2002; Gonyea,

2002; Markides, Eschback, Ray, & Peek, 2007). Poorer economics combined with lower formal educational levels and language and cultural barriers have created a group with significant health issues and limited access to quality health care in this country (Delgado, 2007; Espino & Oakes, 2007; Kim & Lee, 2006; I. L. Martinez & Carter-Pokras, 2006; Trevino & Coustasse, 2007). Their prospects for a healthy older adulthood have been severely compromised, increasing the likelihood of a higher risk for a host of health conditions that will further compromise their well-being.

As this group increases numerically in the next twenty-five years, as discussed in the proceeding chapter, the challenges of meeting their health needs in a culturally affirming or competent manner will only increase dramatically, making the search for new models of health promotion, such as older adult-led, for example, that much more important. Older adults of color are not monolithic in composition, however. Thus, every opportunity to demographically disentangle this group will also be made in the interest of moving the field of health promotion forward in a culturally competent manner, although at times, the reader is warned that this goal will not be possible because of how data are either gathered or reported.

A total of five goals have been identified for this book:

1. provide a demographic profile and projected trends for older adults in the United States with special attention to urban, low-income, and low-wealth older adults of color
2. present the state of the art on older adult health and older adult-led health promotion, nationally and internationally
3. provide the reader with a critical analysis of the rewards and challenges of using an older adult-led health promotion conceptual framework with this population group that builds upon recent thrusts towards civic engagement
4. highlight a series of "high profile," "low profile," and "special population groups" health conditions that will only increase in importance in the next decade and would benefit from a health promotion perspective
5. through the use of a case study and case illustrations (shortened versions of case studies), highlight exemplary "conventional" and "unconventional" programs on older adult health promotion

Each of these goals is noble unto itself. However, in combination they serve as an "engine" that is powerful, dynamic, and highly relevant to both practitioners and academics alike in their quest to better serve the needs of older adults, but particularly those who are urban-based and of color. Although there are older adults of color residing in the nation's rural and suburban areas, urban areas provide a unique context from which to develop health promotion initiatives. The focus of this book will not take away from the importance of rural health promotion, for example. Nevertheless, as the goals state, this book has a particular population group and context in mind, and for that matter, a particular reader, too.

Leviton, Snell, and McGinnis (2000) note that when thinking about urban health promotion in the United States, it is necessary to think of two distinct frameworks. One framework focuses on urbanization; the other is specific to inner-city environments and marginalized groups, and home to probably the greatest health care needs. These two ecological forces provide the depth of understanding on urban health and marginal population groups such as the ones advanced in older adult-led health promotion. Further, Leviton, Snell, and McGinnis (2000) reinforce the point that when health promotion is focused on a city's neighborhoods with the greatest health need, it does not automatically translate into a strengths- or assets-free area. These communities have important assets that must be tapped in any health promotion initiative, including residents themselves. A dramatic shift in paradigms is very much in order, and this will be addressed throughout the remaining chapters in this book.

It is important to ground the reader on how I arguably defined the three most critical key elements of this book: *health promotion, older adults,* and *older adult-led health promotion.* When these terms are interconnected, the definition of each gets altered in a manner that may be totally unexpected yet reflects the reality of the health promotion field and gerontology. The first tends to enjoy the least amount of consensus in the field; *older adulthood* is undergoing significant redefinition based upon the demographic trends of the baby boomers. Finally, the merger of older adult with health promotion and the consumer-led movement (chapter 6) brings a set of values, assumptions, goals, and strategies to the field of health promotion. These terms are dynamic in quality and reflect an ever-expanding view of the key elements inherent in each concept.

Health Promotion: Health promotion draws upon a large number of nonbiomedical disciplines such as psychology, anthropology, education, sociology, economics, philosophy, political science, and social policy, and this represents a strength of modern-day health promotion (Bunton & Macdonald, 2002). However, having many "homes," so to speak, can also mean that health promotion has no one home to call its own.

Cottrell, Girvan, and McKenzie (2002) see health education/health promotion as a cross between a discipline and a profession, and as a result cast this field as an "emerging profession." Health promotion, for the purposes of this book, is considered a profession because of the proliferation of educational programs (undergraduate and graduate) addressing this substance area, the legitimization provided by governments and governmental boards issuing reports on this field, and lastly, because of an increasing body of scholarship on this topic. This is not to say, however, that there is a universal definition this profession is based upon.

It would be an understatement to say that there are many different definitions of health promotion in existence nationally and internationally (McDonald, 1998). There is, as a result, no consensus on how to best define health promotion. Some definitions are highly focused, or some would argue narrow, in view of the intended beneficiaries of the intervention as individuals at-risk; others take a broader community or ecological perspective, and as a result, focus on population groups rather than individuals (Panter-Brick et al., 2006). The approach by Wight and colleagues (2006), which advocates for the increasing of educational attainment among the general urban neighborhood population as a means of strengthening older adult cognitive functioning, is an excellent representation of an ecological perspective. An increase in community educational attainment strengthens the argument of an ecological influence on health by reducing stressful life circumstances and increasing coping among older adults living in low-resource urban neighborhoods.

Some definitions, in turn, have essentially defined "health" in a highly "medicalized" manner; these definitions also see health as medicalized. Definitions of health promotion can usually be divided into two groups: (1) those stressing health promotions goals or ideals and (2) those emphasizing strategies and population target groups (L. Green, Nathan, & Mercer, 2001; Saskatchewan Health 2003). There is no definition of health promotion that enjoys universal appeal. This, incidentally, is not unusual and can be found in other fields that are enjoying rapid growth and influence. Nevertheless, there is a general understanding that any definition of health involving older adults must integrate a functional dimension that results in individualization of the individual. Functional impairment, as a result, cannot be considered a natural consequence of aging (Beck, 2000).

Lewis (2001, p. 1) raises the need for a general consensus on how health and disease get defined: "Yet the terms have no clearly agreed definitions. In fact, the difficulty of defining health has led to most attention being given to defining disease instead." According to Lewis (2001), there are two schools of thought on the subject: (1) the "naturalist" school, which views disease and health as objective entities, and (2) the "normativist" school, which places emphasis on viewing health and disease from a subjective or cultural perspective. These two schools of thought, unfortunately, have not come together because of basic premises and suspicions of each other, making diverging perspectives on health and disease prevalent.

Other definitions of health and health promotion, like the one that follows and those covered in other chapters, take an ecological and policy viewpoint and bring to the field a dynamic conceptualization that both challenges conventional views of health promotion involving older adults and rewards us at the same time. Health promotion, as the reader will soon discover, must be expected to transpire at multiple levels, starting with the older adult individual and rapidly moving along a continuum to include policy-level targets. In addition, health promotion does not have to be restricted to a select number of settings usually associated with older adults and some form of service delivery (McCabe, Hertzog, Grasser, & Walker, 2005; Tagliareni & King, 2006).

L. Green and colleagues (2001, p. 21), stress the need for health promotion to be defined in a manner that takes into account an ecological grounding of health: "The principal definitions of health promotion highlight the importance of policy. Nonetheless, most health promotion initiatives conducted to date have targeted behavior change primarily at the individual rather than the environmental conditions influencing health and health behavior." This ecological perspective has promoted the development of community-based approaches to health promotion that see health and health-related behavior as products of the interdependence between individuals and their social and physical environment (Blankenship, Friedman, Dworkin, & Mantell, 2006; Syme, 2000).

Ecological and policy-oriented definitions of health promotion invariably bring to their definition social and economic justice themes that effectively highlight how social and environmental conditions and circumstances influence health, help-seeking, and health outcomes, particularly for socially and economically marginalized older adults in this society. Health promotion as defined above, I believe, does justice to a field that is increasing in popularity and expanding in influence across a variety of sectors, arenas, and settings (Allegrante, 2006; Buchanan, 2006; Schulz & Northridge, 2004). Further, it captures the importance of the field for addressing the health needs of older adults of color who are marginalized in this society from a broad ecological viewpoint.

Taking a broad perspective may cause concern or anxiety on the part of health promotion professionals, particularly when it comes time to evaluate the outcomes of an intervention. However, taking a narrow or highly focused approach will raise alarms in the community by ignoring obvious social causes of illness, thereby limiting the potential effectiveness of a health promotion intervention. An opportunity for making significant and lasting change in the social circumstances that result in ill health is bypassed accordingly.

Older Adults: Age, not surprisingly, is a social construct that defies being static in definition and is subject to the influence of numerous social, psychological, and health factors and forces. Arriving at a cutoff age for what constitutes "older" is compounded by the interplay of cultural, genetic, environmental, and economic factors (Surbone, Kagawa-Singer, Terret, & Baider, 2006, p. 2): "Old age cannot be understood apart from its context in the lifecycle and from a cross-cultural and historical perspective." Consequently, it is not surprising to understand why extreme social-environmental conditions such as those found in prisons, for example, wield tremendous influence on age-related health conditions that are normally associated with individuals of much greater age.

A number of social trends wield considerable influence on how age is defined, particularly when referring to older adults. Retirement age, for example, is no longer considered sixty-five years of age, depending upon when the baby boomers were born. It can mean sixty-five or sixty-six years. Older adults can be defined in a variety of other ways, depending upon the institution doing the defining. Social Security will have one definition; correctional systems, in turn, will embrace another, yet younger definition as to what constitutes an older inmate (generally fifty years of age). As the reader no doubt concludes, these are two rather extreme versions of a threshold into older adulthood.

This book's definition of *older adult*, in turn, refers to anyone over the age of sixty-five years. However, as addressed in chapter 4, when discussing health promotion, prisons, and older adults and HIV/AIDS, the age group will be fifty years or older. The reader can take issue with the classification of older adults starting at the age of fifty or fifty-five years of age, and that is certainly understandable and expected. However, the discrepancy between these two groups (fifty versus sixty-five years) is due in large part to how the field of corrections views the health of prisoners, and how the field of HIV/AIDS has started to address the longevity of individuals with HIV/AIDS. Both of these fields have come to redefine *older adult* because of social-cultural factors that necessitate a wider view of what age can be considered the beginning of older adulthood because of extenuating health conditions. This definition, however, is much more than an exercise or academic in nature without implications for service delivery, including health. The Centers for Disease Control and Prevention has taken this very viewpoint.

As a result, *older adult* will be defined as anyone over the age of 65 years, with two exceptions: those who are incarcerated and those who are HIV/AIDS positive. It may seem quite unusual to have a definition of *older adult* with such a wide range of age-group onset. However, age and its meaning is a social construct that is influenced by a variety of societal factors and forces. Thus, having context play a critical defining role as to what constitutes *older adult* should not come as any great surprise to the reader. As a result, it is best that I lay out this perspective earlier on in

the book rather than introduce the reader to this viewpoint well into the
book

Older Adult-led Health Promotion: Finally, older adult-led health
promotion combines information from the two previous definitions and
brings a sociopolitical dimension to how these two definitions come to
life, so to speak. A paradigm that has—as a core—consumer-led values,
philosophy, empowerment, self-efficacy, and social actions, brings with
it a unique set of rewards and challenges for both practitioners and
academics alike. Older adult-led health promotion is best defined as an
intervention that has been conceptualized, planned, implemented, and
evaluated, by older adults, the ultimate recipients of these services. This
does not mean, however, that non-older adult providers are not involved
or participating. However, their role as collaborators is dictated by older
adults themselves, and not the other way around.

There are numerous examples of youth-led health promotion, including a book specifically devoted to this form of consumer-led intervention
(Delgado & Zhou, 2008). However, older adults have not benefited from
this concerted attention. Although the definition of older adult-led health
promotion is rather simple in nature, as the reader will see in subsequent
chapters, the premises upon which this definition is based are quite complex and might even be considered revolutionary in thought!

The reader may ask, Is the concept of older adult-led health promotion totally new to this time period? and that is certainly a legitimate
question. The concept of older adult peer-led health promotion is well
over thirty years old, as the reader will see in chapter 5. However, older
adult-led health promotion differs from older adult peer-led health promotion because of the explicit embrace of empowerment and social and
economic justice values. Although empowerment and social justice were
no doubt reflected in the origins of older adult peer counselors, they represented more of a background or implicit understanding rather than the
foreground (explicit), presence in the older adult-led health promotion
model advocated in this book. A shift in paradigms in health promotion
facilitates pluralistic efforts to reach population groups that have historically not been the focus of health promotion efforts, or have not benefited
from initiatives because they failed to take into account the unique circumstances of these population groups (Raphael, 2000). Older adult-led
health promotion represents such a shift in paradigms.

Determining the audience for a book is never an easy task or one that
lends itself to some scientific formula that can arrive at a definitive answer. Who should read this book? It is my hope that this book appeals to

both academics and practitioners alike, as well as the ultimate beneficiaries, the older adult health promoters who will implement health promotion programs. The field of older adult-led health promotion can advance nationally and internationally only if these three worlds come together and collaborate on initiatives and research.

This book, as a result, is intended to draw a bridge between academic, practice, and consumer arenas. However, I am confident that drawing this bridge, so to speak, is a lot easier said than done because these three worlds tend to operate on different principles, use different languages, and march to the beat of different drummers. Further, the "culturally competent" and "consumer-led" approaches advocated by this book make meeting the common needs of these three worlds that much more difficult to achieve. It does not mean, however, that I will not make a noble effort to try. The reader will be the ultimate judge of my success. In essence, this book is intended to appeal to a wide audience with the hopes of bringing together disparate groups in search of a common mission that will benefit society.

This book consists of eleven chapters, divided into four conceptual sections: (1) Setting the Context (four chapters); (2) Health Promotion Theory and Practice (three chapters); (3) Health Promotion Research and Ethics (two chapters); and (4) Reflections from the Field (two chapters). Each of these sections, in turn, seeks to accomplish three goals:

1. ground the reader with the latest developments in the field
2. advance consumer-led health promotion with an older-adult focus
3. provide context in the field with specific attention to urban-based, low-income, and low-wealth, older adults of color

These goals are highly interrelated, although they are often treated as separate entities.

There is little question that the field of health promotion has increased in prominence globally this past decade. Nationally, it, too, has increased in importance and relevance for marginalized, or undervalued, communities. The field of health promotion, however, can only achieve its true holistic potential when it is no longer just the exclusive domain of certain age groups (in this case, the young and the adult population aged up to sixty-five years). Further, the field can ill afford to totally disregard the ravages associated with a history of disadvantage that is often the case in older adults of color living in low-wealth/low-income communities (Ginn, Arber, & Cooper, 2001). The two are inextricably tied together. Health promotion must contend with addressing economic well-being in order to successfully improve health well-being. The area of health promotion and older adults offers the field just as much excitement and adventure as it does any other age population group. This perspective, unfortunately, has not been shared with the same enthusiasm as when addressing the young.

This introductory chapter sought to ground the reader within the subject of health promotion and older adults, and hopefully has done so in a way that both excites and challenges the reader to think of this field from a different perspective. There is certainly no reason why the field of older adult health promotion should not be as exciting as its youth counterpart. This is not to say, however, that the challenges endemic to health promotion are not present when discussing older adults, or that the rewards are any less worthy, just like you would find them within any other age group. Expanding fields such as health promotion should never be restricted as to who should benefit and who should be excluded.

Health is never to be restricted to select groups, and all population groups benefit from a viewpoint that is inclusive rather than exclusive in nature! Health promotion is no different. This is not to deny the challenges inherent in taking this inclusive perspective. However, the alternative is to effectively relegate a significant portion of this nation's population to a second- or even third-grade status regarding heath, an essential element in determining quality of life. Older adult-led health promotion effectively moves older adults into a leadership role and elevates them into prominence. This consumer-led intervention arguably represents the latest chapter in health promotion nationally and internationally, and taps significant demographic trends that will result in research on the potential that older adults bring with them to the field of health promotion.

2

~~~

Older Adult Demographic Profile and Trends

"The United States is on the brink of a longevity revolution. By 2030, the number of older Americans will have more than doubled to 70 million, or one in every five Americans. The growing number and proportion of older adults places increasing demands on the public health system and on medical and social services."

(Centers for Disease Control and Prevention, 2005)

There is an increased recognition of gerontology emerging as a discipline unto itself rather than as a subset of other more established disciplines (Alkema & Alley, 2006; Ferraro, 2006). The emergence of gerontology has been largely fueled by the field's response to a national realization that older adults will constitute an increasingly larger percentage of the country's population in the immediate future. Living in a so-called "aging world" signifies both a major success as well as a major challenge for society (Beck, 2000). Understanding demographic trends without corresponding actions is just an academic exercise and a waste for society, however. This acknowledgment, combined with increased funding and training within graduate schools, has served as an impetus for the field of gerontology.

Social demographics is a topic that many practitioners generally try to avoid because it is often associated with lots of statistics that only academics can possibly understand and enjoy. There are certainly no aspects of social demographics, however, that do not have implications for any form of social intervention, particularly health promotion (Meyer & Wilmoth, 2006). Wilmoth and Longino (2006) stress that diversity among older adults will result in increasing the prevalence of health disparities among subgroups, and necessitate carefully crafting initiatives anticipating demographic trends in the early part of the twenty-first century. Faison and Mintzer (2005), for example, note that it is important that the field of mental health stay relevant to an increasingly diverse aging population. Shah and colleagues (2007), in turn, note that an increase in aging population will project into an increase in the use of emergency medical services, since older adults account for a large proportion of such utilization.

This chapter will specifically focus on demographics and older adults, particularly those who are of color, urban-based, and of low income/low wealth. Every effort, however, will be made to bring this subject to life in a manner that is relevant and more easily digested by the reader. That is the goal of this chapter. The reader who wishes a detailed and in-depth examination of demographics and the aging population in this country will be disappointed, however.

DEMOGRAPHICS, OLDER ADULTS, AND HEALTH PROMOTION

There is a strong association between social demographics and the advancement of older adult health promotion. Koplan and Livengood (1994) almost fifteen years ago drew numerous implications of changing demographic patterns for health promotion and older adults. Hodes (2006) sums up quite well the implication of older people living longer in this country: "Never before have so many people lived so long. Life expectancy has nearly doubled over the last century, and today there are 35 million Americans age 65 and older. The aging of this population—in past decades and in the foreseeable future—presents both a challenge and an opportunity." Health promotion relies upon statistics or qualitative data of various kinds to inform and shape an intervention or project. Inequities or disparities, of illness and treatment, for example, help policymakers, academics, and practitioners decide who is being unfairly treated in this society.

Health disparities among older adults do exist, just like they do for other age groups within the country (Guralnick, 2003):

> Significant health disparities (more illness, more complications) are experienced by most ethnic older adults in the US when compared with their peers in the general population. Heart disease rates are more than 40 percent higher for African Americans than for whites. Latinos living in the US are almost twice as likely to die from diabetes as non-Hispanic whites. The rate of diabetes for American Indians and Alaska Natives is more than twice that for whites. These disparities are believed to result from the complex interac-

tion among genetic variations, environmental factors, and specific health behaviors (p. 1).

These health disparities, as the reader will see later on in this book, necessitate the health promotion field actively seeking to address social ecological (community-wide) factors as opposed to focusing narrowly on risk factors (Stone, Viruell-Fuentes, & Acevedo-Garcia, 2007). Roach (2000) argues that the construct of race, and I would add ethnicity, is not inexplicably tied to health, but racism and poverty certainly are. There are wide differences in poverty rates between older adult subgroups, with African Americans and Latinos having the highest rates of poverty (Biegel & Leibbrandt, 2006).

Robert and Lee (2002) stress the importance and role of community in helping to explain racial differences in health among older adults. Whitfield and Hayward (2003), in turn, argue that health disparities must be addressed within a life-cycle context as a means of better understanding health disparities among older adults. Hummer, Benjamins, and Rogers (2004) raise the alarming conclusion that there is far less understanding on how to eliminate health disparities in older adults, and that there is far more information on how to do this among infants, children, and younger adults. Data gathering limitations severely compromise the development of an understanding of racial and ethnic health disparities among older adults (Maylahn, Alongi, Alongi, Moore, & Anderson, 2005; Sandefur, Campbell, & Eggerling-Boeck, 2004).

Wieringa, Vermeire, Bever, Nelen, and Weyler (2001) found disparities in asthma rates in urban areas for older adults. Arif, Rohrer, and Delclos (2005) found that asthma is a common medical condition among older adult Latino and non-Latino whites. Cortes, Lee, Boal, Mion, and Buttler (2004), in their New York City (East Harlem) study of older adults of color with asthma, identified four key barriers to this group receiving needed services:

1. recognition of the deleterious consequences of asthma on their quality of life
2. high cost of medications
3. non-adherence to the medical regimen
4. difficulty in accessing the health care system

The economic consequences of illnesses have a disproportionate impact on older adults of color when compared to their white, non-Latino counterparts. Kim and Lee (2006), in a unique study of older adult health problems of wealth across race and ethnicity, found that illness had a greater impact on older adults of color. Wealth depletion, however, was far greater upon African-American older adults.

Cattan (2001, p. 11) attributes the upsurge in health promotion and older adults to a realization of how demographic trends will influence society in the not-too-distant future: "Until a few years ago health promotion and older people received at best a fleeting acknowledgement in the pre-retirement courses. Mostly, once older people had reached retirement age the view seemed to be that their health was in steady decline and little could be done to maintain or improve this health status. Recently, however, there has been an increased interest in the promotion of well-being among older people, one of the main reasons being an ageing population." Gross (2008a), for example, examines how projected increases in older adults who have substance abuse problems will increasingly alter how substance abuse services are delivered to this population group, ultimately necessitating residential and outpatient clinics dedicated to those over the age of fifty.

In 2000, 6.6 percent of older adults as a percentage of the population aged twenty-five to sixty-four, were frail, and that is expected to increase to 7.5 percent by 2020, 9.6 percent by 2030, and 10.6 percent by 2040 (Robert Wood Johnson Foundation, 2007). Volland and Berkman (2004), in turn, report on a model for educating social workers to meet the challenges of an aging urban population because of the unique rewards and needs that this group presents, and that their numbers can only be expected to increase in the coming years. The rise in medical efforts to improve the lives of those older adults who are living longer lives is representative of how the fields of medicine and health promotion are being transformed (Hartocollis, 2008).

Older adult demographic trends will only increase the complexities associated with initiating health promotion initiatives and this age group. Kittles and colleagues (2007), for example, raise concerns about using race, a sociocultural construct, as a proxy for measurement of risk for ill health since race represents a complex interaction of biology, culture, and psychological factors. This complexity will only increase as racial and ethnic groups engage in miscegenation and create even greater variations within and between groups in future generations of older adults.

The subject of social demographics, as a result, is one that can play an important role in helping to shape the field of health promotion (Diehr & Patrick, 2003; PR Newswire, 2006b). In regards to older adults, it can provide an important context upon which decisions can be made concerning priorities for types of health promotion initiatives, population targets, and geographical targets, as well as help projects in the future through reliance on demographic trends (Himes, 2002; Wilmoth & Longino, 2006). The Caregiving Project for Older Americans notes that as baby boomers age into older adulthood, it can be conservatively expected that at least 20 percent of them will go without the assistance they need, either through paid or voluntary sources (PR Newswire, 2006b). However, there is no illusion concerning the typical response from practitioners when the topic of demographics is introduced into a conversation. At best, a limited number of "high-profile" statistics will be acceptable. However, an entire chapter on demographics, regardless of the group been addressed, is bound to elicit a quick negative response!

CHALLENGES

The use of demographics to better understand older adults and health promotion, consumer-led or otherwise, is not without its share of challenges, or limitations, that go far beyond representing statistics that are "hard to understand." Although demographics have come a long way over the past few decades, they are still not an exact science, and nowhere is this truer than when discussing undervalued communities that rarely get counted properly for a variety of methodological and sociopolitical reasons. It is rare to have a U.S. Census Bureau report get issued without causing a series of debates about systematic undercounting of racial and ethnic groups. Further, there has been considerable amount of pressure placed on the U.S. Census Bureau to not rely solely on quantitative data gathering methods, since "hard" data methods do not capture the complexities in the lives of the undervalued in our society.

Four dynamic factors influence the percentage of older adults in a geographical area: (1) birth rates, (2) death rates, (3) in-migration, and (4) out-migration. Birth and death rates are probably the easiest to predict. In- and out-migration, however, can prove challenging, particularly in cases where the migration is being done by undocumented residents. States that experience a sustained net gain in out-migration over in-migration generally have higher older adult populations since younger individuals tend to undertake the migration journey, with some exceptions.

Each of the four factors touched upon above is quite dynamic in character, making long-term projections or predictions arduous to accomplish. Nevertheless, projections are possible as long as health promoters are prepared to re-examine their projections and make necessary adjustments as new information becomes available to them.

The subject of newcomer older adults is a case in point concerning obtaining an accurate current profile as well as projecting into the future. In 2002, 7.6 percent of the nation's newcomer population were sixty years of age or older, and 14.4 percent were fifty years or older (Moon & Rhee, 2006). Newcomer older adults, particularly those from non–English speaking countries, have a tendency to underutilize community health services. Developing health promotion programs designed to take into account the unique circumstances of older adults who are undocumented, for example, need to be developed now and for projected population gains in the next two decades.

DEMOGRAPHIC PROFILE OF OLDER ADULTS

Examination of how the older adult population in the early part of the twenty-first century will transform this and other societies is not new, and this potential impact has led to a great deal of discussion or speculation (Diczfalusy, 1996; "Population ageing," 1998). The graying of the country, for example, is not restricted to any one geographical region, affecting rural as well as urban areas (Miller & Dabson, 2005; PR Newswire, 2006b). Further, no state in the nation has been exempt from an increasing percentage of its population growing grayer, too.

As noted in table 2.1, the percentage of the U.S. population aged sixty-five years or older tripled between the years 1900 (4.1 percent) and 2000

Table 2.1.   U.S. Total Population and Population Age 65 or Older, 1900–2060

Year	Population (in thousands) Total	Age 65+	Percent 65+	Percent Increase from Preceding Decade Total	Age 65+
Actual					
1900	75,995	3,080	4.1		
1910	91,972	3,950	4.3	21.0	28.2
1920	105,711	4,933	4.7	14.9	24.9
1930	122,755	6,634	5.4	16.1	34.5
1940	131,669	9,019	6.8	7.2	36.0
1950	150,697	12,270	8.1	14.5	36.0
1960	179,323	16,560	9.2	19.0	35.0
1970	203,212	20,066	9.9	13.4	21.2
1980	226,546	25,549	11.3	11.5	27.3
1990	248,710	31,242	12.6	9.8	22.3
2000	281,422	34,992	12.4	13.2	12.0
Projections					
2020	324,927	53,733	16.5	8.4	35.3
2040	377,350	77,177	20.5	7.5	9.8
2060	432,011	89,840	20.8	7.0	9.6

Note: Data from 1900 to 1950 exclude Alaska and Hawaii. All data refer to the resident U.S. population.
Sources: U.S. Census Bureau publications: Historical Statistics of the United States: Colonial Times to 1970 (1975); 1980 Census of Population: General Population Characteristics (PC80-I-B1); 1990 Census of Population: General Population Characteristics (1990-CPI); Census 2000 Demographic Profile, (www.census.gov/population/www/cen2000/briefs/phc-t13/tables/tab01.pdf); and Population Projections of the United States by Age, Sex, Race, Hispanic Origin, and Nativity: 1999 to 2100 (http://censtats.census.gov/data/US/01000.pdf).

(12.4 percent). The decades between 1920 and the 1950s experienced the greatest increases in this age group. Between 2000 and 2005, it increased by 5 percent (U.S. Census Bureau, 2007). However, the projected increases for the period 2010 to 2020 (baby boomers) will witness significant increases, and older adults will account for 16.5 percent of the total U.S. population, and this will increase to 20.5 percent by the year 2040 (Himes, 2002).

Figure 2.1 provides the reader with a more focused visual representation of how different segments of the older adult population will increase in percentage between the years 2000 and 2050. The oldest of the old (85 years and older), for example, represented 12.0 percent of the total older adult population and is projected to increase to 23 percent, or almost triple in size by the year 2050. Between 2000 and 2005, the oldest of the old increased (20.1 percent) and represented a total of 5.1 million (U.S. Census Bureau, 2007). This age subgroup represents the fastest growing segment of the older adult population, and will bring with it challenges that are similar, as well as significantly different, from those of younger

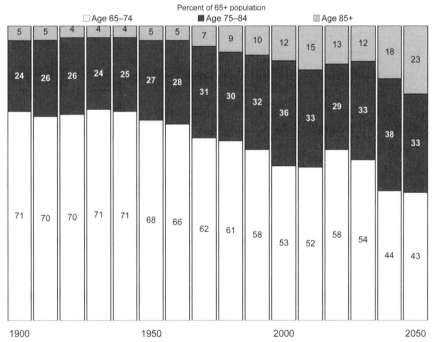

Figure 2.1.   Age Distribution of Older Americans 1900–2000, and Projection to 2050
Sources: U. S. Census Bureau publications: Historical Statistics of the United States: Colonial Times to 1970 (1975); 1980 Census of Population: General Population Characteristics (PC80-1B1);1990 Census of Population: General Population Characteristics (1990 CP1); Census 2000 Demographic Profile (www.census .gov/population/www/cen2000/briefs/phc-t13/tables/tab01.pdf); and "Projections of the Resident Population by Age, Sex, Race, and Hispanic Origin, 1990–2100" (http://censtats.census.gov/data/US/01000.pdf).

older adult age groups (Dunkle & Jeon, 2006). They will number approximately 19 million, or 5 percent, of the total United States population by 2050 (Himes, 2002).

The increased presence of older adults in the population is not restricted to the United States. It was estimated that there were over 400 million people aged sixty-five and older in the world in the year 2000 (Lunenfeld, 2002). It is projected that the world's older adult population will number 973 million by the year 2030, increasing from 6 percent to 12 percent (American Medical Association, 2003). The largest increases (tripling) are expected to occur in developing countries (American Medical Association, 2003).

The importance of disentangling demographic data on older adults must be stressed whenever possible (Lunenfeld, 2002). This is certainly the case in discussing health promotion. The geographical context, for example, plays an important role in shaping the concentration, and/or dispersal, of older adults within communities. LaVeist (2006), however, addresses the need for researchers and policymakers to disentangle race and socioeconomic status, in order to better understand the degree of influence exerted by race disparities due to a function of socioeconomic status. Angel and Angel (2006) go on to note that African American and Latino older adults face disadvantages in achieving "healthful" aging because of social structural inequities. In an earlier study, these authors found that this structural inequality was primarily due to employment history (low-wage) and income (Angel & Angel, 2003). Employment history, incidentally, wields considerable influence on health status because the types of industries that these older adults worked in exposed them to occupational hazards.

DEMOGRAPHIC PROFILE OF OLDER ADULTS OF COLOR

It is not unusual to sit through a presentation on older adults and demographics and develop a very graphic picture of a country that seems to be aging (graying) by the day. This graying of the nation's population has fueled important and often acrimonious debates on a variety of topics, most notably social security. However, it is rare to sit through a presentation where the older adult demographics are disentangled to the point that specific attention is paid to an often-overlooked group such as older adults of color. The complexities of disentangling data notwithstanding, it is necessary to take a specific look at older adults of color in our society.

More specifically, we need to focus on those older adults of color residing in the nation's cities. Angel and Angel (2003), for example, stress the importance of developing a better understanding of older adult subgroups and the importance of eschewing blanket statements pertaining to older adults. Min (2005) advocates for the use of cultural competency as a key element in the practice of social work with older adults of color, and this necessitates a clear understanding of between- and within-group differences. Gonyea (2002), in turn, raises the important point that the diversity of the older adult population will increase along a variety of points beyond the typical and ethnic breakdowns, particularly when discussing newcomers to the United States. However, older adult demographics cannot be separated from the overall demographics of the country. The United States has slowly changed racial and ethnic composition, so that "graying" joins "browning" as a color signifying dramatic population changes in the next fifty years.

In 1990, older adults of color represented 13 percent of the population age sixty-five and older (Pandya, 2005). As indicated in figure 2.2, older

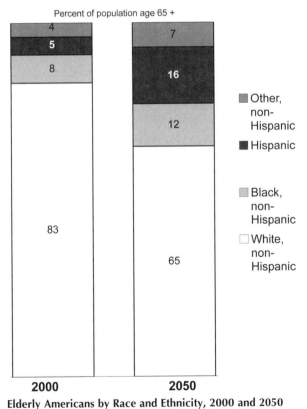

Figure 2.2. Elderly Americans by Race and Ethnicity, 2000 and 2050
Note: The 2000 figures refer to residents who identified with one race. About 2 percent of Americans identified with more than one a race in the 2000 Census.
Sources: U.S. Census Bureau, Census 2000 Demographic Profile (2001); and U. S. Census Bureau, "Projections of the Resident Population by Age, Sex, Race, and Hispanic Origin, 1999–2100" (http://censtats .census.gov/data/US/01000.pdf).

adults of color accounted for 17 percent of the older adult population in the United States in 2000. However, their overall percentage is projected to increase in the next four decades. By 2050, they will represent 35 percent of the older adult population. Among older adults of color, Latino older adults will triple in size between the years 2000 (5 percent) and 2050 (16 percent), making them the largest ethnic/racial older adult group in the country (Himes, 2002). These increases are the result of higher birth and immigration rates within these communities.

In 2005, the nation's people of color totaled 98 million, or 33 percent, of the country's total population of 296.4 million ("Nation's population one-third minority," 2006). The increase in the nation's population was largely fueled by Latinos, the fastest-growing group. This group accounted for close to 50 percent (1.3 million, or 49 percent) of the population growth, and numbered 42.7 million. African Americans numbered 39.7 million, followed by Asians (14.4 million), Native Americans and Alaska natives (4.5 million), and Hawaiians and other Pacific Islanders with 990,000 ("Nation's population one-third minority," 2006). Between 2003 and 2004, the total number of older adults in the United States increased by 351,000, or an average of 7,000 per state ("Bureau estimates," 2005).

OLDER ADULT DISTRIBUTION IN THE UNITED STATES

The older adult population in the United States is not evenly distributed geographically, making reliance on local data significant for the planning of older adult health promotion initiatives. The term "geronitic enclaves," for example, has emerged to refer to geographical areas such as counties that have more than one-third of their population in the older adult category. These geographical areas provide health promotion programs with a concentrated group of older adults, making marketing of such programs easier to accomplish when compared with areas where older adults are not concentrated in a particular area.

Over 50 percent of the nation's older adult population resides in the nine largest populated states, with the Northeast and Midwest regions of the country considered the "oldest" regions based upon the percentage of older adults in their population. In 2004, California, for example, had the highest number of persons sixty-five years or older (3.8 million), followed by New York (2.5 million), Texas (2.2 million), Pennsylvania (1.9 million), Ohio (1.5 million), and Illinois with 1.5 million ("Bureau estimates," 2005).

Nevertheless, a current lack of even distribution does not necessarily translate into a near future or distant future lack of change. There are several states that have recorded significant increases in their older adult population. Some of these states may even surprise the reader because they are usually not associated with having large percentages of older adults. Nevada (4.2 percent) and Alaska (3.8 percent) experienced the highest rate of increase for older adults between 2003 and 2004. Florida, not surprisingly, had the highest proportion of its total population (16.8 percent) consisting of older adults, followed by West Virginia and Pennsylvania (15.3 percent each), and North Dakota and Iowa with 14.7 percent each ("Bureau estimates," 2005).

PROJECTED DEMOGRAPHIC TRENDS FOR OLDER ADULTS

Development of a demographic profile of older adults in the United States serves many worthwhile purposes for health promotion interventions. However, it primarily serves the purpose of developing a projected profile into the near and far future. This information helps society plan for how best to meet the needs of this population group and how it affects society as a whole (Little & Triest, 2001). For example, states with the highest number of older adults also had the highest number of older adults admitted to substance abuse programs, with New York (15,524) having the highest number in 2003, followed by California (7,087), Colorado (4,358), Florida (3,220), and Oregon (2,114) (SAMSHA, 2002). Recent attention has been paid to an increase in the number of older adults who have elected to cohabit with their partners rather than remarry, giving new meaning to how households and family are defined for health promotion purposes (Greve, 2008).

It is important to note, however, that demographic projections are just that, projections. These projections represent the best thinking at the particular time that they are made. Very often, demographic data, when reported, is several years old and can best be thought of as a photographic snapshot in history. As already addressed earlier in this chapter, demographics are shaped by powerful forces such as birth rates, mortality rates, and migration rates (in and out). Each of these rates, in turn, is subject to social influences and events such as disasters. Hurricane Katrina and New Orleans is a fine example of how a natural event can have tremendous demographic consequences involving all humans, but particularly older adults. It is estimated that 71 percent of the victims were older than sixty years of age and 47 percent were over seventy-five years of age (Centers for Disease Control and Prevention [CDC], 2006b). In addition, thousands of individuals/families of all ages were displaced throughout all regions of the country. How many will eventually return to New Orleans after rebuilding occurs is unknown (Ohlemacher & Callimachi, 2006). The number of older adults who will die before relocating back or who elect not to relocate also remains unknown.

An appreciation of demographic trends pertaining to older adults in the United States is best viewed within a worldwide context. For example, it is projected that the number of people in the world aged sixty-five years and older will reach 1.5 billion in the year 2050, with 25 percent of this number being categorized as the "oldest old" (aged eighty years and older), making aging a global phenomenon (Lunenfeld, 2002). The so-called "baby bust" label has emerged to capture the demographic changes occurring in Europe, where there has been a sharp drop in births coupled with a dramatic increase in the older adult population group (Sands, 2005). China, in turn, is also experiencing dramatic demographic shifts, with older adults increasing in representation. In 2000, adults sixty-five years and older accounted for 6.8 percent of China's population. It is projected that this percentage will increase to 14.1 percent by 2025 and 23.6 percent by the year 2050 (Whelan, 2007). Canada, too, has not escaped the graying population phenomenon ("The baby boomers' tab," 2006).

It is projected that by the year 2030, the United States will comprise 20 percent of people sixty-five years or older, representing an increase of 25 percent from 2006 (Dickson, 2006; Fried, 2000). This increase in older adults, however, is not equal across gender. In 2040, it is estimated that for every 100 men sixty-five years or older, there will be 127 women; for those aged eighty-five years and older, the gap increases to 168 women (Administration on Aging, 2004).

It is expected that Latino older adults will numerically pass African-American older adults by the year 2028, when their numbers will reach 15 million (Geronurse Online, 2006). The current and projected dramatic increase in older adults of color will manifest itself differently across states, as already noted. California, for example, will witness an increase from 20 percent of all older adults being of color in 2003, to 41 percent in 2020, or more than doubling in a period of seventeen years (Geronurse Online, 2006). Texas is projecting a 193 percent increase in the sixty years and older group between the years 2000 and 2040, with this group numbering 8.1 million or 23 percent of the total Texas population (Texas Department on Aging, 2003). New York, in turn, will see its sixty years and older population increase by 65 percent between the years 2000 and 2030, from 3.2 million to over 5.3 million. Its eighty-five years and older population, however, will increase even faster (76 percent), from 315,378 to 555,993 (New York State Office for the Aging, 2007).

The 85 and older group, in turn, is expected to triple in size by 2030 (Dickson, 2006). In 1900, it is estimated that only 4 percent of the United States was sixty-five or older, with the average life expectancy at birth at forty-eight years (Fried, 2000). However, by 1997 life expectancy had increased to almost eighty years for women and seventy-four years for men. In cases where individuals lived to the age of sixty-five, however, it can be expected that on average they would live longer by an additional fifteen to seventeen years (Fried, 2000). Consequently, although the older adult population in the United States will witness significant increases in the next few decades, these increases will not be uniform across all older adult subgroups.

The importance of gerontology's responding to changes in demographics and cultural views toward older adults is well recognized (Roth, 2005). These changes, however, involve both the views of non-older adults as well as older adults' views of themselves. In effect, each influences the other in a highly dynamic manner. Nevertheless, there is no denying the critical consciousness raising that must transpire to change how this country views older adults and the potential role they can play in helping to transform this nation.

The future of health promotion and older adults is best viewed and grounded within the context of current and projected demographic trends, as addressed in this chapter. According to the Centers for Disease Control and Prevention (2005), "the United States is on the brink of a longevity revolution" that will have profound transformative powers on the way this society looks in the not-too-distant future and how the health of this nation's population groups are viewed and addressed. Further, as evidenced by this chapter, the nation's older population group will continue to increase in diversity, making generalizations about how to best meet health care needs, including health promotion initiatives, arduous, if not impossible. Developing data that disentangle race and ethnicity in this population group will go a long way toward helping health promotion and other social interventions reach those in greatest need.

Demographic projections are just that, projections. These statistics can be influenced by a host of social-political-environmental factors that can result in higher or lower actual outcomes. Nevertheless, there are some very distinct trends highlighted in this chapter that can only be expected to continue in the next twenty-five years. The nation as a whole will continue to "gray" and "brown," with clear implications for the field of health promotion, among others. The combination of the graying and the browning creates a future scenario that will influence virtually all health care sectors, including the promotion of health initiatives among older Americans, citizens and undocumented alike, as the reader will see in chapter 4 when the nation's prisons are discussed. There, too, will be found the graying and browning of these institutions.

3

≈

Civic Engagement and Older Adults

"In light of contemporary demographic developments, it is hardly surprising that the civic engagement lens has come to focus on the actual and potential contributions of older Americans. By virtue of their emergent numbers, energies, ties, and resources, older Americans stand poised to address myriad individual-level and social problems. This 'reserve army of the leisured' is seen as ready to move."

(Hudson, 2006, p. 13)

The reader may be surprised by the inclusion of the topic of civic engagement in a book on older adults and health promotion, older adult-led or the more conventional approaches. The attractiveness of the concept of civic engagement, as will be addressed in this chapter and throughout the remainder of this book, is that it encompasses particular qualities that are attractive to the fields of gerontology and health promotion, and the concept is enjoying a tremendous amount of currency in all circles, private as well as public. Further, it brings into any discussion civic concepts, such as self-efficacy or empowerment for older adults, making it that much more attractive for social interventions that are consumer centered (Achenbaum, 2006).

The subject of active and meaningful involvement of older adults, particularly when related to volunteerism, has never gone out of vogue in the field of gerontology, as evidenced in the professional literature (D. R. Jones, 2005; Morrow-Howell & Freedman, 2006–07; Romero, Gerrard, & Owen, 2007; Tan, Xue, Li, Carlson, & Fried, 2006). However, the concept of civic engagement in its various manifestations has, too, been the subject of national attention the past thirty-or-so years and more so in the last five years because of baby boomers moving into retirement age. The potential contributions of this growing segment have generated considerable discussion and debate. Consequently, it is not too great a leap, so to speak, to merge civic engagement with a particular age group such as older adults, a social intervention (health promotion), and a social paradigm (consumer led).

Each of these elements brings with it tremendous excitement. However, in combination, civic engagement and older adult-led health promotion offer endless possibilities for innovation, social change, and meaningful participation, or volunteerism, on the part of older adults. For this potential to be realized, it is necessary to broaden our perspective of what constitutes civic engagement and who volunteers across all ethnic and racial groups, and under what circumstances this occurs. Further, there is a need to explore "new" ways of reaching out to communities that have historically not been tapped by social organizations as a volunteer force.

Hudson's (2006–07) assessment of the potential of the "army of the leisured" captures a prevailing view that this country is at a critical juncture pertaining to a large age group ready, and able, to make significant contributions to the nation. However, for this potential to be fully realized, nonprofit organizations and government must be prepared to offer a bold vision of the potential role older adults can play in transforming society and the organizations that serve them (G. O'Neill, 2006–07). This "army" will not stand in reserve very long before they take their energies and commitment and mobilize with or without the aid of organizations. Cullinane (2006-07) provides examples of how civic engagement has been operationalized by some of the nation's leading agency organizations.

The concept of older-adult–driven interventions can certainly find a home in a variety of paradigms, or combination of paradigms. The currency of civic engagement brings forth a potential home for older-adult–driven interventions because this concept is enjoying tremendous popularity in this country and internationally. The concept of civic engagement has increased in popularity in this country in the past five years, although most of this attention has been focused on youth and young adults. Older adults, however, have also benefited from this increased attention, as evidenced by the recent issue of *Generations* that was specifically devoted to this theme, and a book edited by Wilson and Simson (2006a).

There are a variety of ways to ground or legitimize older adult-led health promotion. However, the foundation (values, principles, and theory) surrounding civic engagement represents the most promising national and international well-recognized perspective, or raison d'être, for older adult-led health promotion, and that is why the subject of civic engagement has found its way into a prominent place in this book. The reader, however, may have different ways of bringing older adult-led health promotion to life. That is certainly acceptable from my point of view. The importance, or bottom line, so to speak, is that the older-adult-consumer–led movement progresses in a manner that is affirming and empowering of this population age group.

Civic engagement has effectively emerged as a term that has found wide acceptance among academics, business leaders, and practitioners (Morrow-Howell & Freedman, 2006-07). The currency of this term increases the possibilities of collaboration across disciplines and funding sources. The definition of civic engagement provided by the American Society on Aging (2007) takes the concept of civic engagement and applies it to a specific age group, namely, older adults, and sets a solid foundation for how this term is used in this book:

> Late life civic engagement encompasses actions wherein older adults participate in activities of personal and public concern that are both individually life enriching and socially beneficial to the community. Late life civic engagement can take many forms from individual to electoral participation. A community can be a neighborhood, nation or the world (p. 1).

Thus, civic engagement, according to the American Society on Aging, is varied and benefits individuals as well as their community.

Adler and Goggin (2005) reviewed the literature and concluded that there is no single widely accepted definition of civic engagement. The authors also note that the definition is influenced by a wide range of factors, including age group. McBride (2006–07), in summarizing the literature on civic engagement, notes that there are two distinct "spheres" that are social and political in character. The former consists of actions that effectively connect individuals to each other and generally relate to care or development. Volunteering is usually the most significant in how one of the spheres gets operationalized in the field (Hinterlong, McBride, Tang, & Danso, 2006). The latter, in turn, addresses behaviors intended to influence legislation or electoral or judicial processes related to decision making and resource allocation. Voting typifies this sphere of civic engagement (Galston & Lopez, 2006). Binstock (2006–07) explores the range of impact of political engagement of older adults and their reasons for participation. Martinson and Minkler (2006), in turn, stress the view of civic engagement to include older adults engaged in political endeavors such as racial justice and social justice advocacy. Some theorists, however, would argue that any activity with public consequences can be considered civic engagement, thereby opening up the potential of this concept to be incorporated in a multitude of venues and professions (McBride, 2006–07).

———

Civic engagement is probably best viewed across the life course in order to better understand how it is experienced, the characteristics of those who engage, the community context in which it occurs, and the expectations that go with its varied manifestations (Weiss & Gomperts, 2005). Morrow-Howell (2006–07) argues that the field of civic engagement would benefit from youth and older adults and their advocates, coming together to lobby for more attention and resources to be devoted to civic engagement initiatives. As a result, the importance of civic engagement is too great to be relegated to any one age group in this society. This is not to say, however, that all age groups will share similar goals, expectations, challenges, or barriers to engaging in volunteerism.

Older adults, particularly baby boomers, are not only the fastest-growing demographic sector in the country but are also what is widely considered the healthiest, most vigorous, and best educated older-adult group in the history of the United States (Freedman, 1999). Walker (2001) points out that there has been a transformation of retirement from what can be considered the "elite privileged" to a "mass experience" within the past fifty or so years in Western society. This transformation has resulted in a reconceptualization of what is supposed to happen in this phase of life. Morrow-Howell (2006–07) notes that older adults are a largely untapped national civic resource, particularly when compared with what has happened in the youth service movement nationally and internationally, for that matter.

There certainly is minimal debate about the important role older adults play in this society. R. W. Johnson and Shaner (2005), for example, estimate that the value of unpaid activities by older adults topped $160 billion per year in 2002, or $2,698 per individual. This estimate of volunteering and family caregiving is based upon moderate cost assumptions, too. Unpaid activities by older adults benefit their families and communities, and are also a source of personal fulfillment to other older adults. However, putting a dollar amount on the role of older adult volunteers does a serious disservice to the work that they accomplish in this capacity and is much too narrow in scope, although it is a very popular measure often used to highlight the importance of volunteerism in our society.

Hudson (2006, 2006–07) examines civic engagement involving older adults across the political spectrum and concludes that both the political left and political right understand the tremendous potential of civic engagement and older adults, but each side sees its potential differently.

The potential of civic engagement involving older adults has been heralded as transformative (Reilly, 2006) and as a social legacy of profound importance for the nation (Harvard School of Public Health, 2004). Granville (2001) stresses the relationship between empowerment of older adults and community participation. Empowered participation, according to Fung (2004), helps ensure that public institutions become more "responsive," "fair," "involved," and "effective." Fung (2004), however, argues that with some exceptions, civic engagement scholarship has yet to generate "compelling accounts" of how to reverse the trends of civic deterioration.

Development of a better understanding of who volunteers and the reasons for doing so is a challenge for the field of gerontology (Zedlewski & Schaner, 2006). Cameron (2006) notes that gathering data on civic engagement and older adults has generally focused on white, non-Latinos, thereby limiting our understanding of the extent and nature of volunteering among older adults of color. Freedman (2006–07), in turn, calls for a reconceptualization of the "next stage of work" for older adults to one that can be called the "social purpose work" stage.

Civic engagement, in essence, effectively serves to redefine older adult potential for contributions to their community and to society as whole. This redefinition of potential contribution will have a profound effect across the entire life span for all members of society. Its impact, however, will be far greater among marginalized population groups that have internalized feelings of worthlessness and inability. Older adults from undervalued backgrounds, as a result, can become role models of potential capacity to create positive change. In the case of health and health promotion, this change will alter people's perceptions of how the social environment creates illness as well as health, and empowers them to effect positive change in their lives and the lives of those who surround them.

Civic engagement, as noted by Martinson (2006–07, p. 62), must not be viewed as a strategy to counteract the ravishes of aging: "Civic engagement is being presented as yet another strategy for promoting health among older adults while countering images of decline and loss and addressing societal anxieties about 'greedy geezers.'" This point is very critical in how older adult health promotion gets both conceptualized and implemented. Civic engagement is not a survival strategy for only the "healthy!"

Rissel (1994), like Fung (2004), raises cautions pertaining to the potential of empowerment and how health promotion also applies to the concept of civic engagement. Concerns about a lack of a clear theoretical underpinning, different perceptions on what it means, measurement ambiguities, and structural barriers are important factors in facilitating wide adaptation of civic engagement and older adults. This does not mean, however, that the field must stand by and wait for academics to connect the dots and provide a clear vision for how and when civic engagement can find a prominent place in the field of older adult health promotion. It does mean, nevertheless, that debate and tension can be expected and even encouraged before civic engagement enjoys universal acceptance in the academic and practice arenas.

HISTORICAL OVERVIEW

Civic engagement in American society has been traced back to the beginning of the nation and has been called the core of America's strength by de Tocqueville (Sander & Putnam, 2006). Achenbaum (2006–07) provides a very good overview of the history of civic engagement of older adults in the United States, and notes that it can be traced back almost to the beginning of the nation. The Progressive Era, however, was a particularly significant historical period in fostering civic engagement of older adults. This period was greatly influenced by Theodore Roosevelt's efforts at instituting private–public partnerships to address major national social problems. Roosevelt's strategy, according to Achenbaum (2006–07), built upon three American traditions: (1) fostering voluntary associations, (2) mobilizing political activism, and (3) advancing adult education. Thus, civic engagement and older adults is not a recent phenomenon tied to the emergence of the baby boomer generation; in fact, it predates it by several hundred years.

Twenty years ago, Gardner's (1988) goal of creating a movement of older adults actively seeking to revitalize civil society set in motion the forces that have played a significant role in what came to be known as civic engagement and older adults:

> We believe, without being immodest, that the large numbers of us over age 65 constitute a rich reservoir of talent, experience and commitment potentially available to society. . . . We know the conventional view is that society owes its older citizens something, and we would be foolish to quarrel with that. But we owe something, too, and this is one sense our "operation giveback" (p. 1).

Carlton-LeNey (2006–07) argues that African-American older adults have a long distinguished history of civic engagement in this country that has largely gone unrecognized by the wider society. This legacy lends itself to expanding the potential for African-American older adults to venture out of historically prescribed arenas to new arenas such as those possible with older adult-led health promotion. Latino older adults, too, have a long history of civic engagement within their communities, particularly involving houses of worship. This tradition, unfortunately, has suffered from even greater neglect when compared with their African-American counterparts (Delgado, 2007).

The increased recognition of older adult assets (noneconomical) has converged with an increased recognition of civic participation, to make for a powerful perspective toward this population group (National Association of Area Agencies on Aging, 2007). An assets and civic participation perspective toward older adults is not a new phenomenon, however, and it is well over forty years old. Burnett and Matlins (2006), for example, note that the federal government created two volunteer programs involving older adults as early as the mid-1960s (Foster Grandparents and Retired and Senior Volunteer Program), and established another in the early 1970s (Senior Companions).

BABY BOOMERS AND VOLUNTEERISM

There has been an upsurge in attention pertaining to the swelling of the older adult ranks as the baby boomers slowly arrive at "older adult" status (Rozario, 2006–07). This age cohort brings with it a large base for potential volunteers (Cameron, 2006; G. O'Neill, 2005; Perry, 2007; Wilson & Simson, 2006a; Zedlewski & Schaner, 2006). The potential social contribution of the 77 million baby boomers raises numerous questions about what percentage will actually volunteer, and the nature and extent of this participation (Freedman, 2006–07). Sander and Putnam (2006) note that even if a small percentage of this age group volunteers, their significance can be great:

> Given their large numbers, even modest changes in the boomers' trajectory could have dramatic consequences. All parents and grandparents should hope that these efforts succeed as they will directly shape how civically nutritious a culture and legacy our children and grandchildren will inherit (p. 35).

Interestingly, there has also been increased discussion among strategic thinkers about "Generation X" and the impact this age group has on volunteering as they enter older adult status (Crowley, 2003). Rozario (2006–07) identified age and gender as key factors associated with civic engagement among older adults. Those up to the age of seventy-five report higher rates of participation versus those over this age. Women, in turn, are more likely to volunteer than men. Choi, Burr, Mutchler, and Caro (2007) stress the importance of better understanding formal and informal volunteering among spousal caregiving, particularly examining the role of gender.

This population group has the potential to refine the meaning of older adults (Harvard School of Public Health, 2004):

> The baby boomers will have the opportunity to redefine the meaning and purpose of the older years. As some of the demands of work and family that have commanded their attention in mid-life recede, boomers will have the potential to become a social resource of unprecedented proportions by actively participating in the life of their community. But will they participate? (p. 5).

This question of whether they will participate is one that has garnered the attention of policy makers, practitioners, and academics. The social characteristics of those who will participate, and their motivation and expectations for doing so, as already noted in chapter 2, take on added significance since the baby boomers are not a monolithic group.

Not surprisingly, there is a realization that this demographic shift will bring with it unprecedented demands upon organizations and their ability to respond to the potential that baby boomers bring with them. There is recognition that most programs can only accommodate a very small percentage of older adult volunteers, thereby missing an important resource because of poor planning, and this will require bold new policies to expand the net and make it more inclusive (Gomperts, 2006–07).

Rosenberg and Letrero (2006) raise the multifaceted importance and benefits of volunteerism, and why the United States must maintain or increase volunteer contributions in the future. As baby boomers move into old age, they represent a potential underutilized source for volunteers (Freedman, 1999). Their recruitment and retention, however, cannot be left to chance (St. Paul Foundation, 2007). New initiatives must be mounted to tap this source of energy, creativity, and commitment. Fortunately, significant initiatives are currently underway to both prepare this age cohort for civic engagement and better equip the organizations within which they will play a role (Wilson & Simson, 2006b). It is necessary, however, to pause and note that promotion of civic engagement is not the sole responsibility of government, foundations, and social organizations (Henkin & Zapf, 2006–07). Communities can promote civic norms that encourage voluntarism. When tied to a community capacity-enhancement paradigm, civic engagement represents a viable mechanism for the creation of social good.

SIGNIFICANT CHARACTERISTICS

Reilly (2006), in examining the civic engagement movement among older adults, identifies several significant characteristics that tie this movement to other important social movements in twentieth-century America:

1. a powerful idea that managed to create strong emotion and action
2. leadership that inspired followers and supporters
3. a social-political environment and excellent timing that helped pro-pel an idea onto a national and international stage
4. data to substantiate the urgency of need for action
5. fortuitous timing

Each of these factors separately, but particularly in combination, wield significant influence on how older adults view themselves and how other age groups view older adults.

Hinterlong and Williamson (2006–07), however, do raise possible con-cerns about older adults and civic engagement:

1. Older adults engaging in civic action that only benefits their age group may exacerbate generational tensions.
2. Public opinion about older adults may shift and view them as an entitled group, causing adverse political reactions.
3. Expectations of *all* older adults as needing to be engaged in civic par-ticipation may be unrealistic, leaving those older adults who cannot because of personal circumstances feeling even more misunderstood and undervalued.

Civic engagement must not be thought of as a panacea for all of the ill-nesses confronting older adults in the country. Civic engagement, as a result, is best thought of as part of a comprehensive strategy that actively stresses meaningful engagement of older adults in shaping how these ap-proaches get conceptualized and carried out.

BENEFITS OF VOLUNTEERING

Older adult civic engagement generally serves two primary purposes (Silva & Thomas, 2006): (1) it provides a venue for older adults to engage in productive pursuits and (2) it provides organizations with a no-cost labor force with knowledge, expertise, commitment, and availability. The joy of learning is the third primary purpose that may be implicit in Silva and Thomas's (2006) conceptualization, but it needs to be made explicit. Wilson and colleagues (2006) identify lifelong learning as a critical factor in civic engagement, one that can be effectively utilized as a motivator for recruitment and retention of older adults. Narushima (2005), in turn, points to the transformative mechanism embedded in community volun-teering for older adults. In essence, older adult civic engagement is best conceptualized as a win-win situation with the volunteer, organization, and society benefiting from this activity.

Hinterlong and Williamson (2006–07), for example, identify the potential social bridge role of civic engagement bringing disparate age groups together. The American Society on Aging (2007, p. 2) points out the potential benefits that older adults bring to society: "Our whole society benefits when older adults, with their will developed from a lifetime of experience, are given opportunities to further get to transmit their skills and perspectives through initiatives based on their strengths."

Greene and Cohen (2005) note that a resiliency perspective serves to enhance specific survival skills to assist older adults to cope with difficult personal and social situations. Benefits derived by older adults are not restricted to just working with adults or other older adults. Fried and colleagues (2006), for example, report on the gains of older adults participating in a volunteer program in elementary schools. Older adults' physical, cognitive, and social activity increased, suggesting multiple benefits from volunteering.

The social, psychological, and health benefits of volunteering by older adults are well recognized in the field and can cover a wide variety of spheres such as general health (W. M. Brown, Consedine, & Magai, 2005; Morrow-Howell, Hinterlong, Rozario, & Tang, 2003; Thoits & Hewitt, 2001; Van Willigen, 2000), delayed mortality (Harris & Thoreson, 2005), protective factor (Greenfield & Marks, 2004), physical and mental health (Greenfield & Marks, 2004; Lum & Lightfoot, 2005; Schwartz, Meisenhelder, Ma, & Reed, 2003), sense of belonging and connectedness (W. M. Brown et al., 2005; Okun & Michel, 2006), and general well-being (Morrow-Howell et al., 2003), to list but a few areas. Choi (2007), in a study of older adult volunteer instructors and their peer teaching experiences, found peer teaching of older adults to be a complex phenomenon. However, mutual shared experiences combined with mutual contributions and role reversal (instructor and student) enhanced learning by both peer educator and student.

Last, the opportunities for older adults to utilize their competencies and knowledge as community leaders open up new vistas for this age group. This broadening of civic engagement opportunities to include positions of leadership in these efforts, as evidenced by older adult-led health promotion, benefits both older adults and communities (Corporation for National & Community Service, as quoted in Eccleston & Priestman, 2007, p. 4):

> To attract Baby Boomers to volunteering, experts on aging agree that non-profit groups and others must boldly rethink the types of opportunities they offer—to "re-imagine" roles for older American volunteers that cater

to Boomers' skills and desire to make their mark in their own way. This is vitally important to ensuring that the potential of this vast resource is tapped to its fullest.

Creation of a cadre of older adult leaders in community efforts represents the natural extension of a community capacity-enhancement perspective on civic engagement, and one that holds a bright future for this movement.

BARRIERS TO VOLUNTEERING

McBride, Sherraden, and Pritzer's (2006) qualitative study of low-income and low-wealth families and civic engagement found that engagement is taking place, but there are substantial obstacles to doing so. Their find-ings are not surprising for anyone who has worked with these types of families, and the findings are applicable across the life span to include low-income and low-wealth older adults. McBride (2006–07), in a study specifically focused on civic engagement and older adults, raised im-portant questions of concern about those adults for whom this form of participation has historically and currently been inaccessible. Older adults with disabilities or compromised health may face exclusion; a large population group with an important perspective is thereby left out, and is also not able to draw on many of the benefits, as noted above, that go with active and meaningful civic participation. Institutional capacity can be increased to encompass a broader spectrum of who should be engaged in the multifaceted venues for civic engagement.

Reilly (2006) strikes an optimist note in declaring that a national trans-formation has begun for organizations to engage older adults in activities with social good goals. This transformation has resulted in a de-emphasis on a perspective (deficit) that views older adults as consisting of needs, to one that is asset-based and views older adults as entering a period of enhanced capacity, personal renewal, and intellectual growth. The emer-gence of a "wellness" concept to characterize programs stressing health rather than illness is such an example. Achenbaum (2006), however, issues a call for creation of new roles and opportunities at the commu-nity level for older adults. Older adult-led health promotion is a direct manifestation of an assets paradigm involving this population group and represents an "innovative" approach toward civic engagement.

C. Johnson, Parel, Cobb, and Uy (2003, p. 5), too, raise concerns about the need for serious action and initiatives to create and expand meaning-ful opportunities for older adult civic engagement. However, a new vision for older adult participation is coming into contact with the realization that community-based organizations' capacity to absorb them is seriously lacking: "To the extent that this is already happening throughout the nation, federal and local governments, foundations, and corporations must quickly direct significant resources towards developing model programs and initiatives that support the engagement of older adults." This challenge may be simpler to raise than to address in the field. Ignoring it, however, will not make it go away.

Finally, Gonyea and Googins (2006–07) view the subject of older adult civic engagement from a different perspective, calling for expanding the boundaries of what is typically considered corporate volunteerism. The corporate sector has been considered "slow" in offering employees greater flexibility in their work and retirement options, thereby limiting the civic contributions of employees and their corporate employers.

INCLUSION VERSUS EXCLUSION

As already noted, the concept of civic engagement was never meant for any particular age group, although it certainly has found a home among the young and adults. Hudson's (2006) observations pertaining to the importance of diversity raises this very point:

> Because of their historical experience with economic discrimination, social isolation, and political marginality, older women and older populations of color are more likely than their white male brethren to bring critical extra-aging concerns to the civic arena. Broad participation will better reveal the diversity of civic concerns older people carry with them (p. 16).

Diversity of civic concerns is certainly one of the primary benefits of broad participation among the older adult group (McBride, 2006–07; St. Paul Foundation, 2007). However, the position that all older adults can provide for others, regardless of individual challenges, forces the field of health promotion to examine the varied ways that assistance can be provided, and how this is accomplished can inform the field. Boerner and Reinhardt (2003), for example, in their study of support provided by older adults who were disabled, showed that there are feasible ways support can occur, even in situations where the individual providers are in need of assistance themselves. The potential for expanding civic engagement to all older adults, regardless of functional abilities and needs of their own, is exciting.

There are significant challenges in applying civic engagement to older adults. Nevertheless, there are even more challenges when discussing what barriers older adults of color face in formally volunteering:

1. lack of transportation (Cameron, 2006; O'Neill & Lindberg, 2005; St. Paul Foundation, 2007)

2. financial needs (Hudson, 2006; McBride, 2006–07; St. Paul Foundation, 2007)
3. lack of English language skills (Fong, 2006)
4. legal status in the case of the undocumented (Crowley, 2003; Delgado, Jones, & Rohani, 2005)
5. lack of awareness about opportunities and benefits of volunteering (McBride, 2006–07)

Each of these challenges is noteworthy, and they take on greater significance in combination with each other.

Not unexpectedly, low-wealth/low-income older adults of color bring with them a view of health that has been shaped by a life history of discrimination, classism, and sexism. This operative reality is both to be expected and addressed in older adult-led initiatives such as health promotion. After all, the construct of diversity helps ensure that there are multiple realities to contend with and none is more important than the others. Their perceptions of what constitutes health and what are the "acceptable" and "expected" benefits from participation necessitate clear articulation of the vision that will guide older-adult health promotion and to what extent it encompasses the experiences of undervalued older adults.

EMPOWERMENT AND SOCIAL JUSTICE

Although the concept of empowerment is a central feature to how civic engagement becomes operational, it often gets done implicitly rather than explicitly in any discussion of the virtues of older adult civic engagement. Empowerment and social and economic justice constructs represent a central feature, or tenet, of older adult-led health promotion, as they should in the more conventional health promotion approaches (Squire, 2001). Story (2007) sums up the close relationship between empowerment, social change, and public health and health promotion quite well:

> Principles of empowerment and social change are paramount to the success of public health programs. Assessing needs, recognizing barriers, developing change strategies, and making a plan of action facilitate the eventual occurrence of social change. This social change can also be initiated by policy change, and in any case it is a result of action by individuals, groups, organizations, cultures, and/or society.

The close relationship between empowerment, social change, and health promotion will also be addressed in chapters 5 and 6.

The bringing together of empowerment and social justice serves to cast civic engagement in a particular light that influences the selection of the most appropriate strategies to achieve equity for older adults from undervalued backgrounds. Wallerstein and Freudenberg (1998) a decade ago effectively linked health promotion and social justice and concluded that these two concepts address the role of power and the importance of empowerment in creating a state of well-being for marginalized groups.

Holstein (2006) comments on the potential leadership role that older adults can play in society and in helping to achieve social justice goals for the nation:

> The old ought to become moral entrepreneurs, to take leadership roles in exemplifying commitment to the community and to social justice. They had the time, experience, etc., to play roles that others did not. Today, I have serious questions about that recommendation. I trust, indeed hope, that people will choose those roles but I no longer believe that it ought to be held up as an expectation. . . . What we all need is respect and recognition, which our society has been so closely tied to work-related roles and, for women, also to appearance (p. 25).

Holstein's charge, so to speak, places older adults front and center in the nation's quest to tap social capital in service to the country.

CIVIC ENGAGEMENT AND OLDER ADULT-LED HEALTH PROMOTION

The close association between civic engagement and health promotion as conceptualized in this book provides academics, practitioners, and older adult volunteers with a rationale for coming together in pursuit of common goals. Older adult-led health promotion provides a viable avenue for engaging older adults in new roles that capitalize on their knowledge, time, and commitment for making important contributions to their community and society in general. Mind you, there are countless other avenues for older adults to become involved in their communities. Nevertheless, having them play active and leadership roles in a health promotion initiative represents an innovative and important venue for their engagement.

Civic engagement and older adults must be conceptualized as consisting of many different items on a menu, so to speak. Not every older adult will be interested in health promotion. Some will find intergenerational work involving school children and reading, for example, as the most meaningful way for them to contribute. Others, in turn, may find helping small business owners develop their businesses to be their preference. Older adults should not be limited in how they want to contribute to their community based upon a very limited menu. They should have viable choices across an entire spectrum of venues. Civic engagement and older adult-led health promotion, too, must provide a wide range of options and not be limited to one or two types. Health promotion is a very broad field, and no aspect of this field should be considered off-limits to older adults.

Reilly's (2006, p. 7) challenge for civic engagement can easily be applied to older adult-led health promotion: "In order for the civic engagement movement to progress from success to significance, to become a major significant social change event of the 21st century, a coordinated multi-sector response is needed." A multi-sector response, such as the one being proposed in older adult-led health promotion, represents a viable approach within the health promotion field. If civic engagement is to take hold in a meaningful manner among older adults, and at no time is this more relevant than when discussing consumer-led health promotion, older adult leadership must play a prominent role in these efforts (Manning, 2006).

The potential of older adults leading health promotion initiatives is very much dependent upon organizations in a position to sponsor these interventions being willing, and able, to do so. Endres's (2005) research on nonprofit organizations' preparedness to use older adults as volunteers found them unprepared. Having older adult volunteers take on leadership roles further raises questions of organizational capabilities. The Gerontological Society of America's (O, Neill & Lindberg, 2005, p. 1) first priority issue of a report on civic engagement of older adults recommends to "modernize the nation's senior and civic service programs." Older adult-led health promotion responds well to this and other challenges by older adult-focused professional and practitioner organizations.

One way of facilitating the engagement of older adults is to make available a standardized training curriculum that will cut down on the costs associated with training older adult volunteers. In the health promotion arena, Schneider, Altpeter, and Whitelaw (2007), undertook a meta-analyses of ten national evidence-based or best practice health promotion programs for older adults that systematically utilized older adult volunteers and explored the feasibility of a generic training program for volunteers. The authors concluded that such a training program is feasible and can contribute in multiple ways toward the goals of promoting healthy aging. The importance of providing training to older adult volunteers is recognized in the field of health promotion. No older adult can be expected to be proficient in all aspects of health promotion, and a similar conclusion can be applied to professional staff, too.

Huang and colleagues (2002), in a study of the effectiveness of health promotion educational programs among older adults in Taiwan, found

these programs to be quite effective in improving health-related knowledge and behaviors among those aged sixty-five to sixty-nine years old,
married, having higher formal educational levels, and living with family. This demographic group may well represent the most "attractive"
audience from a health promotion perspective. Nevertheless, modifying
interventions to take into consideration the social context of the older
adult participant is a fundamental principle of effective older adult health
promotion, regardless of the demographic profile of the older adult group
being targeted.

The emergence of civic engagement as a goal for all age groups in this
country has brought with it excitement and the potential of contributions
from all older adults, and not just those who are physically healthy and
sufficiently wealthy to volunteer. The construct of civic engagement, like
any other social construct, is fraught with challenges as well as rewards
for the fields of gerontology and health promotion. Nevertheless, the
continued growth of the older adult ranks as the nation's baby boomers
enter retirement age must not be ignored by policy makers. However,
their engagement in civic actions will require bold new ideas about how
best to tap this reservoir of talent.

As the reader has no doubt realized, civic engagement is operational
based upon the social circumstances of the older adult contemplating
volunteering. The worldview and priorities of older adults with histories
of being undervalued by society will differ with their counterparts who
have been privileged. This observation, incidentally, is not unique to
older adults. Nevertheless, there is no escaping the fact that marginalized
older adults suffer from multiple sources of discrimination, such as race,
gender, income, and, in a high number of cases, various forms of disabilities, along with ageism, a new form of discrimination. These social
circumstances must weigh in on how civic engagement can reach out to
include these groups of older adults. Civic engagement and health promotion represent a natural alliance, particularly when health promotion
is older adult-led, as discussed in the following chapters of this book.

Rozario (2006–07) rightly observes that predicting the future of volunteerism among older adults is difficult because of the potential interplay
of numerous social, economic, and political forces. Nevertheless, there
is no controversy about the importance of this nation being able to tap a
largely untapped reservoir of talent or social capital found among older
adults. Also, there is no argument about the need and importance of
new perspectives and models of older adult civic engagement. It is important to end this chapter on civic engagement on a note that says that

not every older adult must participate in civic ventures to be "worthy," as commented by Martinson (2006–07, p. 64): "Finally, the option of not being involved in civic engagement as an older adult must be honored." It is important, however, to provide "genuine" and "meaningful" opportunities for all older adults who wish to engage in volunteerism. This fundamental belief will provide options for older adult groups that have historically not been available to them.

4

⟋⟍

Older Adult
Health Care Needs

"As a greater number of people reach old age, medicine is challenged to develop new approaches to this population. Health promotion, not just treatment of disease but improving the quality of life for older persons, must play a role."

(Fried, 2000, p. 1)

Addressing current and projected health care needs of older adults, and particularly those who are low income/low wealth, urban based, and of color, is bound to be a daunting task for any author, just like it is in the field of practice (Policy Research Associates, 2006). Dynamic changes in population, combined with the emergence of new research findings specific to this population age group, is compounded by the increased diversity found among older adults of color. This does not mean that the field is not capable of meeting these challenges. However, it does mean that the level of awareness and sophistication that is needed pertaining to health promotion and older adults, particularly those of color, must be heightened, along with flexibility and innovation in the design of health promotion initiatives intended on reaching this population group. Anything short of such an effort fails to maximize the potential of health promotion reaching and helping this population group (Lang, Lawry, & Anderson, 2005).

Loprest and Uccello (1997), for example, raise concerns about uninsured older adults over a decade ago. Not unexpectedly, the sixty-five-years-and-older uninsured group is largely composed of Latinos and African Americans/blacks in this country (Doty & Holmgren, 2005;

Okoro, Young, Strine, Balluz, & Mokdad, 2004). Fronstin (2005) goes on
to note:

> While 65.1 percent of the non-elderly population is white, whites comprised
> 48.1 percent of the uninsured. Individuals of Hispanic origin were more likely
> to be uninsured than other groups (34.3 percent). . . . This may be due in part
> to the fact that 52.4 percent of the Hispanic population reported income of
> less than 200 percent of the federal poverty level. Also, a higher proportion of
> Hispanics are immigrants and may work for small firms or be employed on a
> part-time or part-year basis. However, even at high income levels, Hispanics
> generally were more likely to be uninsured than other racial groups and were
> less likely to have employment-based health benefits (p. 1).

Health promotion initiatives targeting the uninsured older adult group,
as a result, take on tremendous prominence, particularly when these
older adults are clustered in certain geographical areas of cities.

The value of immunization for older adults is probably the least controversial form of health promotion because of their costs and effectiveness
in preventing deaths in this age group, and it is another example of how
older adult profile influences health promotion (Karuza, 2001). Lifetime
nonreceipt of immunization against influenza or irregular vaccination
among older adults is considered a critical factor in making older adults
more vulnerable to a range of illnesses. Sambamoorthi and Findley (2004),
however, found that a significant proportion of older adult Latinos (43
percent) and African Americans (45 percent), when compared with white
non-Latinos (28 percent), had never received influenza immunizations.
Gallagher and Povey (2006), in a study of older adult intentions to vaccinate against influenza based in England, advance a theoretical model
for better understanding, facilitating, and hindering determinants, with
implications for health promotion.

A number of researchers have issued the challenge or sounded the
alarm to the field that older adults of color face current and future serious health issues because of their life circumstances (Committee on
Population, 2004a,b; Fronstin, 2005; Gold et al., 2006; Jackson & Knight,
2006; Kelley-Moore & Ferraro, 2004; Stewart et al., 2006). Race, ethnicity, gender, income and wealth, and urban context, are all key factors in
shaping the health status of older adults of color. Older adults of color,
for example, have disproportionate rates of morbidity and mortality from
chronic diseases, such as blood pressure, cancer, heart disease, diabetes,
depression, anxiety, and obesity (Center on an Aging Society, 2004). The
proportion of adults age fifty and older with chronic health conditions
among older adults of color is quite high, with African Americans (77 percent) having the highest proportion and Latinos (68 percent) having the
next highest percentage (Center on an Aging Society, 2004; Singal, 2006).

Asian Americans, in turn, have the lowest percentage (42 percent) and are also lower than white non-Latinos (64 percent).

It is a challenge, however, to be able to examine older adult health care needs without forgetting that this population group also possesses incredible strengths and assets. Birkhead, Riser, Mesier, Tailon, and Klein (2006, p. S2), although specifically addressing youth assets, note the implications of this perspective for other groups: "The approach of focusing on assets and positive attributes in addition to risk may also be beneficial in addressing other public health problems in other population groups." The mere fact that these individuals have managed to surmount a tide of trials and tribulations associated with oppressive forces in this society is a testament to their resiliency and assets. Those older adults of color who died along the journey, unfortunately, did not possess the assets and social navigational skills of their counterparts who managed to survive and even thrive.

This chapter will be divided into three major health-related categories: (1) high-profile health needs, (2) low-profile health needs, and (3) special population group needs. The first addresses health needs that enjoy a good degree of attention in the field as evidenced by the literature and invariably get mentioned by both practitioners and academics when discussing older adult health care needs (Schoeni, Freedman, & Martin, 2005). The second category, in turn, refers to older adult health needs that have not received the attention they deserve. This does not mean, however, that this will always be the case. It does mean that low-profile older adult health needs have not benefited from the funding, research, and scholarship that high-profile health needs have received in this country. Finally, the last category on special population groups attempts to highlight the importance of three subgroups (the homeless; gay, lesbian, bisexual, and transgender; and prisoners) that generally get overlooked when discussing health promotion and older adults. These three groups represent a growing demographic trend and present the health promotion field with a host of unique challenges (because of their social circumstances) that counterparts without these circumstances do not.

The reader may disagree with the classification of some of these health needs as either high- or low-profile, or with special population groups selected, and that is to be expected. For example, Burbank (2006) specifically identifies five groups of older adults that are particularly vulnerable and thereby at increased risk for unhealthy consequences: (1) the incarcerated; (2) the homeless; (3) gays, lesbians, bisexuals, and transgenders; (4) those with HIV/AIDS; and (5) the frail. The reader will notice that three of these five groups fall into the special groups category in this book and the other two fall into the high-profile and low-profile groupings.

The classification of health needs is very much a judgment call on my part. The reader, in addition, may take issue with some "missing" health needs, such as breast cancer, oral health, hearing and eye impairments, arthritis, and pain, for example (Herr & Decker, 2004; Kiyak & Reichman, 2005; Oliver-Vazquez, Sanchez-Ayendez, Suarez-Perez, Velez-Almodovar, & Arroyo-Calder, 2002; Song et al., 2007). The presence of pain increases with aging, and how it gets manifested and experienced differs as well. When pain goes untreated or is poorly managed, it can result in older adults experiencing cognitive difficulties and reduced activities of daily living (Davis & Srivastava, 2003). The lack of space has necessitated that certain needs, such as pain, either not get mentioned or only get mentioned in passing without due justice being done to them.

Further, high-profile, low-profile, and special population groups of older adult health needs will be covered in a general overview manner as a means of providing the reader with a grounding and appreciation of how certain types of older adult health needs are viewed and addressed in the field of health and health promotion. Each of the health issues touches upon data related to the importance of the condition and highlights several challenges for the field, as well as examples of health promotion efforts. Each of these health conditions is worthy of one or a series of books based on its importance. Consequently, this chapter highlights why these health conditions and special population groups are high-priority areas for older adult health promotion, and it sacrifices depth in order to achieve a higher degree of breadth.

These health conditions can also be found in other age groups, but their interactions with older age groups bring an added set of challenges. In reality, there is a tremendous amount of overlap between these categories, and the grouping of needs can be subject to debate, which is understandable. Viewing these health needs from a narrow perspective denies the social context in which they occur. Nevertheless, my primary goal in covering this material in this particular manner is to make it user friendly and provide the reader with a substantial foundation upon which to develop or facilitate health promotion initiatives. Every effort will be made to point out the interaction of these health needs with each other and how comorbidity brings with it a set of challenges for health promotion and the need to take a comprehensive view of older adult health needs rather than a highly focused, or specialized, perspective.

HIGH-PROFILE HEALTH NEEDS

Diabetes

There are certainly numerous perspectives that can be taken to examine diabetes. The financial costs of diabetes, for example, can be extremely high. In 2002, it was estimated that the financial costs to the country were $132 billion, of which $92 billion was in direct medical costs and $40 billion in indirect costs such as disability, work loss, and premature mortality (National Diabetes Information Clearinghouse, 2005).

It is estimated that the number of older adults over the age of sixty-five with diabetes in the United States is 18.7 percent (American Medical Association, 2003; DeCoster & George, 2005). The seventy-five years and older cohort, however, is projected to have the highest increases in diabetes between the years 2000 (1.2 million women and 0.8 million men) and 2050 (4.4 million women and 4.2 million men) (American Medical Association, 2003). It is estimated that approximately 40 percent of adults between the ages of forty and seventy-four, or 41 million people, have a prediabetic condition that increases the risk for type-2 diabetes (National Institutes of Health, 2005).

In 2000, diabetes was the sixth leading killer in the United States and was responsible for over two hundred thousand deaths each year (CDC, 2001). This can be translated into a twice-the-risk factor for people with diabetes when compared with counterparts without diabetes (National Diabetes Information Clearinghouse, 2005). Further, diabetes and high blood pressure are closely correlated, with 73 percent of adults who have diabetes also having high blood pressure (National Diabetes Information Clearinghouse, 2005).

Diabetes, as already noted in chapter 2, is disproportionately found among people of color, particularly African Americans and Latinos (Henry J. Kaiser Family Foundation, 2005). However, Native Hawaiians are 2.5 times more likely to be diagnosed with diabetes than their white, non-Latino counterparts (CDC, 2001). Among Latinos, there is considerable risk for type-2 diabetes that is almost twice as high (1.9 times) as white non-Latinos. Among Mexican Americans, however, the risk is two times higher (CDC, 2007c; Kaushik et al., 2007). It is estimated that two million Latinos currently have diabetes, while 60 percent are overweight, increasing their chances for contracting diabetes (Heller, 2007).

Environmental hazards (air pollution and extreme heat) can worsen the health of individuals with diabetes, and this is particularly the case with older adults, particularly those living in urban areas of the country (Environmental Protection Agency, 2007). It should be noted that African Americans (2 times) and Native Americans (2.6 times) have higher rates of diabetes-related complications such as kidney diseases and amputations (CDC, 2007c).

More than 10 percent of the Latino community has diabetes, and it is also estimated that one-third of them are undiagnosed (PR Newswire, 2006a). Almost 21.4 percent of Latinos aged sixty-five and older have been diagnosed with diabetes (NOVA, 2004), with almost 15 percent of all

Mexican Americans having diabetes (Pearsey, 2007). However, diabetes among American Indians and Alaska Native populations is considered the highest in the world, with more than 50 percent of this population group having this illness, and its prevalence is still increasing (Roubideaux et al., 2004). One study of Native Americans in Arizona, for example, found diabetes to be the most common among older adults, with rates as high as 74 percent among women (sixty-five to seventy-four years of age), raising serious alarm among public health professionals.

Diabetes also can be found disproportionately in cities (Fountain, 2006; Kleinfield, 2006a,b), and adherence to treatment regimen also differs accordingly. Rhea and colleagues (2005), for example, in a study of barriers to diabetes education in urban patients, found that a host of socioeconomic factors wield considerable influence on perceptions of barriers to participating in health education programs. Holder (2001, p. 204) notes that beliefs of African-American older adults concerning being overweight as an indicator of good health make health promotion efforts targeting diabetes quite challenging: "Negative beliefs may decrease this motivation and promote a more fatalistic attitude leading to decreased dietary adherence." The family, however, has been identified as a key social support in helping African-American older adults to a diabetic regimen that is effective.

The prevention and early intervention in diabetes is well recognized in the field. A small reduction in weight and an increase in physical activity are effective in reducing the risk of diabetes for older adults. Lifestyle interventions can reduce development of diabetes by up to 71 percent among older adults (National Institutes of Health, 2005). However, lifestyle health promotion interventions must be based upon a solid understanding of sociocultural context and how it influences diet and exercise. Lack of cultural congruency and involvement of significant people in the older adult social network will meet with minimal effectiveness, at best (Fustes, 2002).

Hypertension

Heart disease and stroke are considered major health problems within communities of color. Davison and colleagues (2007) note that among Latinos, for example, these illnesses are considered the leading cause of mortality among men (27.1 percent) and women (32.2 percent). The economic consequences are far reaching, with an annual estimate of costs for cardiovascular disease at $163 billion by the year 2050. Thus, to say that hypertension is common among adults aged sixty years and older would not be an understatement (Kostis, 2004).

It is estimated that almost 50 percent of all persons over the age of sixty years have hypertension, making older adults at risk for a range of severe health consequences (Rigaud & Forette, 2001). However, it is estimated that fewer than approximately 25 percent of older adults with high blood pressure are receiving adequate care (Kostis, 2004). Hypertension is a health condition that has serious consequences if left untreated. Among older adults, hypertension is considered a fairly common condition that significantly increases morbidity and mortality risk. Lloyd-Jones, Evans, and Levy (2005), in a study of hypertension among the oldest of the old (eighty years or older), found that 70 percent had hypertension and fewer than 10 percent had normal blood pressure levels.

Adherence to antihypertensive therapies, in turn, is considered to be low, increasing the importance of effective health promotion initiatives on the topic, particularly in the case of older adults whose first language may not be English and whose cultural values and beliefs may make complementary and alternative medicine more attractive than conventional medical approaches (Bell et al., 2006). In similar fashion to other health needs covered in this chapter, African Americans report higher rates of hypertension than white non-Latinos or Latinos. Rhoades and Buchwald (2003), in a rare study of hypertension among older urban Native American primary care patients, found the prevalence of diagnosed hypertension to be 38 percent, and equally troubling, the possible undiagnosed hypertension to be 23 percent.

Hypertension does not transpire within a cultural or emotional vacuum. Consequently, health promotion efforts seeking to reduce hypertension among older adults must take into account a context to increase effectiveness of interventions. In one study based in Japan, for example, researchers found that older adults who lost a loved one but believed in a "good afterlife," were less likely to experience hypertension when compared to those who did not believe in an afterlife (Krause et al., 2002). Ostir, Berges, Markides, and Ottenbacher (2006), found a strong relationship between high positive emotion and lower blood pressure among older adult Mexican Americans. Hajjar, Frost, Lacy, and Kotchen (2006) examine hypertension and older adults from the perspective of health care provider beliefs in healthy behaviors. The authors found that those providers with positive beliefs were better able to convey these beliefs to older adults, increasing the likelihood of helping them adopt positive health behaviors that reduce hypertension, such as exercise and proper nutrition.

This context, in turn, influences help-seeking practices as well as efforts to self-medicate. Neafsey (2001), in a study of older adults attending a blood pressure clinic, found that 86 percent of the 165 subjects reported taking at least two self-medications, creating an adverse reaction. Self-medication, as a result, takes on greater significance in the case of older adults with low health literacy levels and those relying on cultural-based medications. The implications for health promotion efforts to both better understand self-care practices and develop interventions that are grounded within a cultural context is self-evident, just like it is with the other health needs addressed in this chapter.

Depression and Other Mental Health Needs

The mental health needs of older adults, including those of color, are increasingly being recognized in the gerontological field, particularly the major barriers that must be surmounted (Choi, 2005; Massanari, Barth-Jones, Chapleski, Mahlmeister, & Smitherman, 2002). It is estimated that 70 percent of all primary care visits by older adults result from some form of mental health need, such as generalized anxiety, depression, somatization, stress, or adjustment disorders (American Psychological Association, 2003). However, it is also estimated that 63 percent of older adults do not receive the treatment they need. The percentage of older adults with depression who do not receive adequate treatment is even higher, at 75 percent (American Psychological Association, 2003). Studies suggest that only a very small percentage of older adults (3 percent) actually report seeing a mental health specialist for their needs (American Psychological Association, 2003). It is not unusual, for example, for depressed older adults to have visited a general physician in the month prior to committing suicide, with 20 percent having seen a doctor on the same day and 40 percent within one week of a suicide (Brody, 2007).

Older adults' not viewing or presenting their needs and symptoms as being mental-health related has complicated the process of screening, diagnosis, and treatment. Inadequate screening has resulted in older adult mental health needs going undiagnosed and untreated for extended periods of time, if at all, and this stage in the help provision process is increasingly being identified as critical in the mental health of older adults. Harris and Cooper (2006), not surprisingly, stress the importance of better screening and treatment of depression among older adults living in the community. Arean and Unutzer (2003), in turn, found that oldest of the old, low-income adults of color experience inequities in depression management and raise barriers related to access to preferred treatments that are culturally grounded. However, Kales and Mellow's (2006) review of the literature on racial differences in the diagnosis and treatment of late-life depression concluded that physician bias based upon patient race did not explain all diagnostic and treatment differences. Williams and colleagues (2007) studied older adults who were poor and had a diagnosis of dementia and found that those who lived alone were less likely to be diagnosed by their primary care physician than those who had active caregivers.

The topic of Alzheimer's disease is one that probably most often comes to mind in the general public when discussing older adults and mental health in this country. However, it is not restricted to the United States, as Canada, for example, also struggles to address the needs of an increasingly older adult and ethnically diverse population (Luh, 2003). Alzheimer's disease is closely related to age, particularly among the oldest of the old. Two older adults out of 100 aged sixty-five have Alzheimer's. However, by age eighty-five, the number increases to thirty to thirty-five out of 100 (Wygant, 2007). Health promotion efforts that delay the onset of this disease by six or more months will have tremendous implications for the field of health promotion (Clevenger & Quinn, 2007). Lack of information on Alzheimer's that targets older adults of color has been identified as a key barrier in having them play more assertive roles in getting the aid that they need (Ayalon & Arean, 2004).

Alzheimer's strikes Latino older adults at an earlier age (67.6 years) than their white, non-Latino counterparts (74.6), making the importance of delaying the onset of this disease even greater among Latinos (Berger, 2005). C. M. Clark and colleagues (2005) conclude that the mean age for symptom onset for Latinos is 6.8 years earlier when compared with white non-Latinos. A low formal education level, combined with high rates of vascular disease, particularly diabetes, increases the risk of Latinos contracting Alzheimer's at an early age when compared with other groups (Elliott, 2001).

Older adults with inadequate diets can manifest a range of cognitive, emotional, and behavioral symptoms, which can eventually result in mental illness. Valcour and Paul (2006) address the emerging mental health (dementia) problems associated with HIV and older adults, particularly the impact of long-term, highly active antiretroviral therapy and immune reconstitution. The combination of HIV, advanced age, and cognition is not fully understood and has tremendous implications for health care delivery.

Love and Love (2007) note that screening for mental health problems among older adults is generally not routine in health promotion programs that are community based. Proper nutrition, as a result, has both physical as well as psychological benefits (Chernoff, 2001a,b; McCabe-Sellers & Johnston, 2006). Ostir and colleagues (2006), as reported earlier in the previous section of this chapter regarding hypertension, found a strong association between high positive emotions and lower blood pressure among older Mexican Americans (average age of 72.5 years old), increasing the relevance of health promotion programs that are nonpharmacologic in focus. Prince and colleagues (2007), in a review of the literature on mental health, found that depression increases the risk for the onset of type-2 diabetes.

There are certainly a variety of approaches that health promotion programs can take toward addressing the mental health needs of older adults. Health promotion programs that stress physical activity, for example, have been found to not only improve physical health but also improve the mental health of older adults (Lautenschlager, Almeida, Flicker, & Janca, 2004). Health education campaigns that provide older adults with a better understanding of mental health symptoms and destigmatize treatment open up the field for innovative efforts, particularly among older adults of color.

Health promotion programs focused on improving and preventing the onset of emotional problems among older adults, like the other health conditions raised in this chapter, must endeavor to ground these interventions within the cultural context, definition, and interpretation of the older adults being targeted (Cattan & Tilford, 2006). Early intervention takes on prominent importance in the case of older adults and Alzheimer's disease because of the early onset of this disease and older adults of color.

Injuries from Falls

The association between falls and older adults is quite strong in the minds of the general public. Commercials graphically describing an older adult who has fallen and unable to reach a telephone have probably been seen by countless millions of people in this country. Consequently, there are few practitioners and academics who would not list injuries resulting from falls as one of the key needs in the field of gerontology because of the serious health consequences that can result from these events (Holmes, 2006; Pynoos, Rose, Rubenstein, Choi, & Sabata, 2006). The multitude of health consequences resulting from falls makes prevention of falls among older adults a high priority area for health promotion (Allen, 2001). Not surprisingly, the importance of health promotion programs specifically targeting falls has only increased in the past decade and will no doubt continue to show greater prominence in the next decade.

Falls among older adults not surprisingly are considered one of the major causes of hip fractures and hospitalization in the United States. Stevens (2006), in an analysis of unintentional falls among older adults sixty-five years of age or older from 1993 to 2003, and from 2001 to 2005, found that this is a common occurrence among almost 30 percent of this age group on an annual basis. The average hospitalization for older adults with hip fractures was almost a week (Popovic, 2001). Baker (2001) notes that falls in the home after hospitalization of older adults seventy years or older occur with 14 percent of patients within the first month after hospital discharge. It is estimated that as many as 20 percent of hip fracture patients die within a year of their injury (Leibson, Toteson, Gabriel, Ransom, & Melton, 2002). In 2004, 14,900 older adults died from injuries involving unintentional falls, 1.8 million were treated in emergency departments, and 433,000 were hospitalized (CDC, 2006a).

Like other health conditions covered in this chapter, there are significant differences between gender, race, and ethnicity. Falls were higher among men (46.2 per 100,000) than women (31.1 per 100,000). Rates also differed based upon race and ethnicity for men: white non-Latinos, 48.3 per 100,000; Asians and Pacific Islanders, 35.6 per 100,000; African Americans, 22.3 per 100,000. White non-Latinas had the highest rates among women with 32.8 per 100,000; Asians and Pacific Islanders, 23.2 per 100,000; and African Americans, 13.9 per 100,000.

The financial costs of unintentional falls can be considerable, with an estimate of $200 million for fatal medical costs and $19 billion for nonfatal injuries. Nonfatal falls' medical costs are $12.6 billion (63 percent) for hospitalization, $4 billion (21 percent) for emergency department visits, and $3 billion (16 percent) for treatment in outpatient settings (Finkelstein, Chen, Miller, Corso, & Stevens, 2005; Stevens, Corso, Finkelstein, & Miller, 2006). The CDC (2007a) estimates that the average cost of a fall is $19,440, not including doctor's services. The financial costs are higher among older adult women when compared with men since they account for almost 80 percent of all fractures (Stevens & Olson, 2000). Women are responsible for 72 percent of all hip fracture hospitalizations (National Centers for Health Statistics, 2006). One estimate of future costs puts the figure at $43.8 billion (in current dollars) by the year 2020 (Englander, Hodson, & Terregrossa, 1996).

Health promotion efforts targeting older adult unintentional falls generally are multipronged in nature: (1) exercise programs such as tai chi and yoga, (2) medication reviews to reduce their side effects and interactions, (3) eye examinations, (4) improvement of lighting in the home, and (5) reducing hazards in the home (CDC, 2007a; Tummers & Hendrick, 2007). Some of these approaches will entail that health promoters collaborate with practitioners of other disciplines, such as fitness experts (Marzilli, Schuler, Willhoit, & Stepp, 2004). Health promotion, as a result, can involve some or all of these approaches and can transpire in a wide variety of settings, community as well as institution based.

Obesity and Overweight

A disproportionate amount of attention will be placed on this section because of how weight is closely tied to a variety of other health problems addressed. The impact of being either obese or overweight is widely accepted as a major national problem, with the United States accounting for one-third of the world's fifteen-and-older population that is either overweight or obese (B. Johnson, 2006). Since 1991, rates of obesity have increased at a dramatic pace among all adults in the United States, widely considered to be at epidemic proportions. However, it is likely to have a disproportionate impact among older adults because of the challenges associated with introducing new diets and potential mobility limitations restricting physical activities (Flood & Newman, 2007; Center on an Aging Society, 2003).

Mortality resulting from obesity in the United States, for example, is disproportionately found among older adults (Flegal, Williamson, Pamuk, & Rosenberg, 2004). Growing trends in obesity have resulted in increases in diabetes among older adults and corresponding illnesses such as kidney infection, glaucoma, cataracts, and peripheral neuropathy, for example (Francoeur & Elkins, 2006). Recent estimates have obesity (BMI equal to or greater than 30) and overweight (BMI equal to or greater than 25) at rates of 33 percent and 67 percent respectively among adults (Evans, Renaud, Finkelstein, Kamerow, & Brown, 2006). It is estimated that over 50 percent of all African-American/black women between the ages of twenty and seventy-four years are obese, compared with 31.5 percent of white, non-Latina counterparts (Pearsey, 2007).

Like most health conditions, being obese or overweight is generally the result of the interplay of poor eating habits and sedentary lifestyles across all age groups, and not just among older adults. Physical exercise, for example, is absent in the lives of a significant portion (40 percent) of older adults, with only 10 percent participating in any form of "vigorous" physical activity (Cohen-Mansfield, Marx, Biddison, & Guralnik, 2004). There are, not surprisingly, gender, socioeconomic, and racial differences for the levels and types of exercises that are considered acceptable (N. W. Burton, Turrell, & Oldenburg, 2003). Chernoff (2001a,b), in turn, argues that nutrition has an important role in health promotion and older adults.

Health-related conditions resulting from obesity can take on great significance when discussing older adults. Georgetown University's Center on an Aging Society (2003), in a report titled *Obesity among Older Americans: At risk for chronic conditions*, notes:

> Obesity not only affects the health of older adults, it also affects their day-to-day lives. Older people who are obese report more activity limitations and more feelings of sadness and hopelessness than those who are not obese. Differences between obese and non-obese populations are particularly striking for people age 51 to 69 (p. 1).

Symptoms of depression (sadness, worthlessness, and hopelessness) can accompany obesity among older adults.

The subject of obesity is one that can be addressed as a separate entity. However, its close relationship to other subjects such as smoking and depression, for example, necessitates that it be viewed within a broader context from a health promotion perspective (Friedman & Parekh, 2007; Roff et al., 2005). This section, however, will attempt to treat this subject as a separate entity for the purposes of facilitating discussion, although this is certainly not the way life is, so to speak.

Being obese or overweight brings a series of health consequences that result from these weight conditions, and these consequences are not restricted to youth or the young adult population in the United States (Firdaus, Mathew, & Wright, 2006). There is general agreement that the amount of people who are obese or overweight is reaching an epidemic proportion in the United States (W. D. Evans et al., 2006). Burton (1999) undertook a review of the literature on determinants for physical activity initiation and maintenance among older adults living in the community and concluded:

> Not surprisingly, participation in physical activity declined with increasing age, increasing disability, incident health conditions, poor self-rated health, and symptoms of depression. Factors that favor an active lifestyle include being young, white, male, married, having a higher educational level, no emotional distress, overall better health and less disability (p. 1).

Zedlewski and Schaner (2006) highlight the importance of older adults remaining active and engaged in helping to ensure better health. In their review of the literature on older adults and volunteering, they concluded that those who volunteer not only live longer, but are also better physically and mentally than their counterparts who do not volunteer. Zedlewski and Schaner (2006, p. 1) note: "Boomers' volunteerism could benefit society, boomers themselves, and potentially, government. But a better understanding of who is volunteering today should precede efforts to support volunteerism among aging boomers." Bopp and colleagues (2007) advocate for the use of spirituality, culturally specific activities, and the use of social support within the church as a means of encouraging physical activity such as walking, for example.

There are numerous challenges in health promotion efforts addressing poor eating habits and limited physical exercise among older adults. An increase in physical activity is often a key element in a large number of health promotion programs targeting older adults, particularly among older adults of color (Firdauset al., 2006; Hui & Rubenstein, 2006; Struck & Ross, 2006; Wilbur, McDevitt, Wang, Dancy, Briller, Ingram, et al., 2006). Attempts to create health promotion programs that are physical-activity focused have proved fruitful. Gordon (2004), for example, notes the prevalence of cultural stereotyping as a major impediment in the creation of physical activity programs targeting older adults of color. One study of television viewing and pedometer-determined physical activity among adults of color found that average daily television watching was associated with reduced pedometer-determined physical activity levels (Bennett et al., 2006). Increased television viewing is associated with lower physical exercise among youth of color, too.

Resnick, Vogel, and Luisi (2006), in a pilot program with a primary goal of increasing motivation among older adults of color, concluded that the theory of self-efficacy lends itself to encouragement to exercise, particularly when grounded within a culture-specific content. Self-efficacy is considered one of the strongest predictors of physical exercise across socioeconomic groups of older adults (Clark & Nothwehr, 1999). Wolf and colleagues (2006) describe the use of tai chi training on physical performance and hemodynamic outcomes among frail older adults. Adler and Roberts (2006), too, advocate for the introduction of tai chi as an activity for improving the health of older adults and note that this form of exercise is "slow" and "gentle," and thus particularly suitable for older adults with chronic illnesses.

Schuler, Roy, Vinci, Philipp, and Cohen (2006) conclude that there are few studies that have examined ethnic differences in motivation and barriers to exercise among older adults. Belza, Walwick, Schwartz, Shiu-Thornton, and Naylor (2004) examined facilitating and hindering factors for older adults of color engaging in activities that promote physical exercise. They found that a number of factors can be successful in facilitating exercise, such as fostering relationships among participants, offering programs at residential sites, involvement of the families of older adults, collaboration with local social service organizations, provision of transportation, and ensuring physical safety. These facilitating factors can be grounded within a language/cultural context as a means of addressing both structural and social barriers to participation.

Wyman (2001) notes that probably one of the greatest challenges facing the health promotion field is how to motivate those older adults who are habitually sedentary to participate in regularly scheduled activity or exercise training programs. There are, however, highly creative ways of introducing physical activity to older adults. For example, the introduction of an organized game called "granny basketball" in Cedar Rapids, Iowa, provides older adult women with physical activity that is also recreational and social (Borzi, 2007). Six-on-six games, as part of the Granny Basketball League, consist of women in their fifties and sixties in organized activities that introduce social as well as physical activities. One participant noted, "If we win, bonus. If we don't, let's have fun" (as quoted in Borzi, 2007, p. C23). In Harlem, New York City, a synchronized swimming group of adults aged fifty and older called the Harlem Honeys and Bears, started in 1979, is another innovative effort. Participants practice every day and are attracted to this club as a result of health concerns, but social interactions also play an important role in maintaining membership (Robinson, 2007). These two forms of activity may not be feasible for older adults who have various forms of disabilities that limit their participation in organized activities. However, health promotion and physical activity must be conceptualized along a continuum from low functioning to high functioning. This opens up the possibility for physical exercise to occur in different forms, depending upon the circumstances of the older adult.

There is general agreement that health promotion efforts to increase physical activity must be based upon a broadening of the context, or socioenvironment, to increase exercise among older adults. Health promotion strategies that include physician advice and monitoring and evaluation by a professional were found to be important among 70 percent of all participants in one study (Cohen-Mansfield et al., 2004). However, several factors or considerations were also important, such as easy access (close location), types of exercises, cost, and social comfort (similar in age to other participants), making it essential for health promotion efforts to take into account the perspectives and expectations of participants. Health promotion programs such as Urban Motion: Movement and Music for Health, based in Calgary, Canada, an eight-week program consisting of a one-hour dance followed by one hour of socializing, combine fun, exercise, and socializing, a powerful combination in any form of older adult health promotion program (G. Harris, 2006).

Bickmore, Caruso, and Clough-Gorr (2005) report on a novel program that tests the acceptance and viability of an animated conversational agent that targets urban older adults of color. An animated agent serves as an exercise advisor that interacts with participants through a touch-screen computer provided as part of the study. A relationship ensues that enhances participation in daily walking. The use of computers to reach older adults in their homes represents one of the latest advances in the use of technology to reach those who may have difficulty leaving their homes to attend health promotion programs. The costs associated with technology, however, must be weighed when computers and the Internet must be made available as part of the intervention in the case of older adults with low-income/low-wealth. Telewalk, a combined cognitive and behavioral intervention, is another example of a health promotion program to increase physical activity (walking) among older adults (Kolt et al., 2006). This project is a home-based telephone motivational counseling intervention that has shown positive results in New Zealand.

Finally, it is important to end with a challenge to the field of health promotion, not to focus on obesity and overweight on an individual level, which would create prejudice, or blame the victim (Cohen, Perales, & Steadman, 2005). A focus on the "O" word (obesity) shifts the causes of this condition from an ecological (social and economic) perspective to an individual lifestyle preference perspective. Increasing availability of healthy foods in local supermarkets and schools, or campaigns to promote walking, for example, typifies an ecological approach.

LOW-PROFILE HEALTH NEEDS

As noted earlier in this chapter, but certainly of significant importance to be worth repeating, low-profile health needs among older adults, particularly those of color, are still significant health needs for this population group. The term *low profile* does not signify low importance or minimal consequence. Rather, it signifies low awareness on the part of policy makers, practitioners, and academics. The low-profile health needs that follow will hopefully not remain out of the nation's consciousness, and may eventually receive the recognition they deserve. This recognition translates into additional funding for research, service provision, and training, and moving these health needs to high-profile status.

HIV/AIDS

The subject of infectious diseases is one that is invariably associated with various forms of stigma and immorality, and this is certainly the case when discussing sexually transmitted diseases such as HIV/AIDS. Health promotion efforts to eradicate these diseases or treat them once they are contracted cannot ignore the influence of morality and how it shapes public opinion and policy in the United States, regardless of the age of those who are infected. The first reported case of older adults with AIDS appeared in 1984, when three cases of AIDS in patients over sixty years old were presented and attributed to late diagnosis because testing was not done until late in the progression of their illness (Inelman, Gasparini, & Enzi, 2005). In what is probably the latest documented case, an eighty-two-year-old in Washington, D.C., was diagnosed with HIV ("Birds, bees and HIV for seniors," 2007). Nokes (1996), in one of the earliest books on HIV/AIDS and older adults, raised the need for society to shift its views on broadening the category of who is at risk for contracting HIV to include older adults.

A dramatic shift in prognosis for HIV-positive persons has resulted in longer life expectancy (Kaiet al., 2006; Nichols, Speer, Watson, Watson, Vergon, Vallee, et al., 2002). It was estimated that by the beginning of 2001, there were more than 60,000 individuals with HIV/AIDS over the age of fifty years. However, Kai and colleagues (2006) note that the prevalence is likely to be underestimated because of delayed screening and recognition of the disease. Inelmen and colleagues (2005) reached similar conclusions, and note that 10 percent of HIV infection is found in adults over the age of fifty, and this may be an underestimate of risk because few people in this age group routinely get tested. Hickey (2006) echoes a similar theme about the failure of policies to target those over the age of fifty, and a similar conclusion can be drawn about health care workers ignoring the potential of HIV in this age group. It is projected that 50 percent of the nationally prevalent AIDS cases will consist of older adults by the year 2015 (Valcour & Paul, 2006), bringing a new dimension to any discussion concerning health promotion and older adults in the United States.

The topic of HIV/AIDS is no longer one that is exclusively associated with youth and young adults (R. Baker, 2005; Emlet, 2004a; Inelmen et al., 2005; Kohi, Klein et al., 2006; Neundorfer et al., 2004). It is estimated that one in six people with AIDS in the United States is at least fifty years or older (Mack & Ory, 2003). Over 10 percent of new AIDS cases in the United States transpire in people over the age of fifty (Health Watch, 2002). More specifically, AIDS among African Americans aged fifty years or older accounted for 11 percent in this racial group through 2000 (Health Watch, 2002). In Puerto Rico, those over the age of sixty years account for 3.9 percent of all AIDS cases reported through March 2004 (Santos-Ortiz, Matte, Correa-Nivar, & Pintado-Diaz, 2004).

The topic of HIV/AIDS, as already noted in the introductory chapter, is one that is usually reserved for youth and young adults and rarely has been associated with older adults. However, this absence, or neglect, has done a serious injustice to this population group and the field of health promotion because it effectively eliminated a population group from consideration of interventions meant to prevent HIV infection (Bassey, 2003; Emlet & Poindexter, 2004; Joyce, Goldman, Leibowtiz, Alpert, & Bao, 2005; Sheth, Moore, & Gebo, 2006; Szerlip, DeSalvo, & Szerlip, 2005).

Poindexter and Keigher (2004), however, advance the notion that there has been tremendous progress on knowledge and older adults with HIV/AIDS since this initial period. The subject of HIV and older adults, for example, was of sufficient importance and concern that the National Association of Social Workers (2003) issued a publication titled *The Aging of HIV* because of the increasing numbers of older adults, and particularly those of color and the impact of this disease on their communities. Older adult women, for example, are at particular risk for contracting HIV during intercourse when compared with younger women. This is the result of reduced vaginal lubrication and thinning of vaginal walls (estrogen loss) and a weakening of the immune system.

Sexuality is not supposed to be a topic that applies to older adults, and therefore the possibility of contracting HIV and other STDs is nonexistent. A relatively recent study counters this argument and finds that older adults well into their sixties and seventies do engage in sexual activities on a regular basis (Carry, 2007). Peale (2004) raises the misconceptions nurses may have about older adult sexuality and the important role that sexual health promotion can play in enhancing the lives of older adults. Pangman and Sequire (2000), in turn, specifically address the subjects of sexuality and the chronically ill older adult from a social justice perspective. The authors stress the potential role of health promotion for helping address the devaluing of sexuality among older adults by society, and respecting the rights of older adults and helping them to promote social justice to enhance their quality of life through health education, counseling, and support. In 2007, New York City's Department of Aging initiated sex education classes for older adults, and New York City's City Council earmarked $1 million for HIV education and older adults ("Birds, bees and HIV for seniors," 2007).

Davies (2001) touches upon the role and importance of sexuality among older adults and why the topic is rarely addressed in the professional literature on health promotion with this population group. However, with the increased numbers of older adults contracting various forms of STDs, including HIV, this topic will only increase in visibility in the near future, particularly in older adult retirement communities and areas of the country where older adults are prominent in numbers. Canada, too, is beginning to address the prevalence of HIV among older adults. It is estimated that 10 percent of those testing positive for HIV are over the age of fifty years ("Birds, bees and HIV for seniors,"2007).

Goodroad (2003) identified older adults as a group that society does not perceive as being at risk for contracting HIV. However, this group is not only at risk for contracting HIV but also for contracting a host of other diseases that further comprise treatment of HIV. Fritsch (2005) identifies the formidable barriers this group must surmount to receive services that are age specific in a world that associates HIV/AIDS with youth. Winningham, Richter, Corwin, and Gore-Felton, 2004, in turn, raise the importance of older African-American women gaining greater awareness of their vulnerability to HIV through intimate partner sexual relations. Emlet (2004b) and MacLean (2001), too, raises challenges in meeting the needs of this age group. Older adults with HIV may not feel comfortable seeking spiritual support from religious institutions that they belong to, thereby limiting support to close family and professionals (Poindexter & Emlet, 2006). Willard and Dean (2000), and Vance and Robinson (2004), stress how the interaction of the aging process affects HIV among older adults.

The impact of HIV on older adults goes far beyond health and social factors and enters into the financial realm (Keigher, Stevens, & Plach, 2004). Older adults, particularly older adults of color when compared with white, non-Latino older adults, are more likely to possess fewer economic resources (Joyce et al., 2005). Crystal and colleagues (2003), too, have arrived at similar conclusions. Older adults of color have generally gone through a different exposure route (drugs and needle sharing) when compared with their white, non-Latino counterparts.

Interestingly, D. R. Brown and Sankar (1998) almost one decade ago recognized the challenge of HIV/AIDS in aging communities of color and the implications this population group has for health care delivery, health promotion, and caregiving by family. Smith, Levy, and Schensul (2002), in a study of attitudes of older adults of color toward people with HIV/AIDS, found that contrary to stereotypes, they did not have negative attitudes, particularly in cases where higher HIV knowledge, family presence and level of education, and lower religiosity were prevalent.

Coon, Lipman, and Ory (2003), and Goodkin and colleagues (2003), note that social and behavioral HIV/AIDS prevention interventions focused on older adults are sorely lacking, particularly in the development of a better understanding of risk-taking behaviors. Ageism, according to the authors, is the primary barrier to development of these age-specific interventions. Coon and colleagues (2003), however, observe that the field of HIV/AIDS must not neglect the lessons learned from work with younger population groups but must consider important intervention lessons learned from work with older adults in other health arenas. Outreach and education campaigns have played an important role in helping to prevent HIV among other at-risk population groups. However, lessons learned, with requisite modifications to take into account the social context of age, can still find success with older adults. Schrimshaw and Siegel (2003), too, have identified ageism as one of the key barriers for older adults with HIV/AIDS getting the support and the attention they warrant.

Shippy and Karpiak (2005), argue that older adults with HIV/AIDS are largely disconnected from informal supports and must, as a result, rely upon formal caregivers. Orel, Wright, and Wagner's (2004) research on state department of public health literature targeting older adults and HIV/AIDS, however, found that only fifteen out of fifty states had such publications. The importance of making HIV information age specific is greater when discussing a population group that has low literacy overall, and particularly in health matters (Orel, Spence, & Steele, 2005). Hammond and Treisman (2007) raise concerns that the diagnosis of depression among older adults with HIV/AIDS is a serious challenge in the field because symptoms such as fatigue, decreased appetite and sexual urges, and poor memory are also symptoms that appear in those individuals with HIV. One New York City study of older adults with HIV, for example, found that they were thirteen times more likely to be suffering from depression when compared with cohorts without HIV (Marcus, 2006).

Scandlyn (2000), in an analysis of when AIDS went from an acute to a chronic disease, notes that AIDS, like most chronic diseases, carries a stigma. This stigma, in turn, can be compounded by cultural factors, too. Further, having a chronic illness tends to place increasing responsibility on those who have the illness to care for themselves. This onus takes on greater significance when the individual with the chronic illness has very limited external options to get assistance because of sociocultural factors such as race/ethnicity, income, documented status, and limited English-speaking language skills.

Not surprisingly, AIDS-related deaths among African Americans fifty-five years of age and older (17.00 per 100,000) were almost sixteen times that of white non-Latinos (1.1 per 100,000), and almost fourteen times that of Latinos (3.1 per 100,000) in this age group. AIDS, as a result, is the third leading cause of death among African Americans ages forty-five to fifty-four and fifty-five to sixty-four, respectively (Health Watch, 2002).

African-American women, who are estimated to represent an increasingly higher percentage of all known AIDS cases as age increases, accounted for 21 percent of AIDS cases among fifty- to fifty-nine-year-old women, 22 percent for ages sixty to sixty-four, and 25 percent for those over the age of sixty-five years (Health Watch, 2002). African-American women, as a result, account for 48 percent of all known AIDS cases for women over the age of fifty-five, compared with 34 percent for white non-Latinas and 17 percent for Latinas through the year 2000 (Health Watch, 2002). HIV is the fifth leading cause of death among African-American women aged fifty-five years or older, higher than the seventh leading cause for African-American men in the same age group (Health Watch, 2002).

Increased survival rates for HIV-infected persons have played a significant role in the steady increase of older adults with HIV/AIDS in the past decade (Kohli et al., 2006). Increased survival rates, however, are not totally responsible for the increased number of older adults with HIV, and it would be a serious mistake to think so (Altschuler, Katz, & Tynan, 2004; Williams & Donnelly, 2002). New cases of HIV/AIDS diagnoses among the forty-five-years-and-older age group have also shown an increase (Kohli et al., 2006). This increase makes the importance of prevention for this age group that much more significant.

G. Brown (2002) notes that the problem of HIV/AIDS among older adults has not received the recognition it deserves because of stereotyping, lack of prevention strategies targeting this age group, misdiagnoses, and a general lack of research. Further, health history taking rarely involves asking questions about drug use in the past. Thus, older adults with histories of injection drug use, for example, may have put themselves at high risk for HIV, and since they are no longer doing so, may not think of themselves as possibly being HIV positive. Older adults with HIV/AIDS experience stigma that severely limits their access to needed services. The lack of age-specific programs and services further limits their access (Fritsch, 2005). Creation of public information campaigns that target older adults of color, and do so within a cultural and language context, are very much needed. Poindexter (2004) recommends increasing resources for older adults with HIV. However, increased attention must stress the importance of support, stigma, and social activism to increase resources.

Driver Safety

Old age is a period that is often associated with numerous losses that can have a profound impact on well-being. However, giving up the "right" to drive an automobile is probably one of the most controversial topics related to driver safety and older age, and is a topic that rarely is considered when discussing losses associated with aging (Adler & Rottunda, 2006; Bedard, Stones, Guyatt, & Hirdes, 2001; Carr, Flood, Stegar-May, Schechtman & Binder, 2006; Rudman, Friedland, & Chipman, 2006; Transportation Research Board, 2004). Although the subject of older adult driver safety is a national issue, it has particular relevance for older adults living in areas of the country with inadequate public transportation systems, rural as well as urban. In cities where unmet transportation needs exist, loss of a driving license can result in reduced well-being (Peck & Hess, 2007).

The upsurge in older adult population addressed in chapter 2 has resulted in the number of licensed drivers age sixty-five or older to increase by 17 percent between 1994 and 2004, compared with 13 percent for the total number of licenses issued during this period (CDC, 2007b). Consequently, statistics related to older adult mortality and accidents must be viewed within this context, in order to better understand why driver safety is a health promotion topic worthy of attention. Older adult injuries and fatalities from motor vehicles are very high. In 2004, according to the CDC (2007b), there were 3,355 deaths of older adults resulting from motor vehicle accidents. Older adults over the age of eighty have the highest crash fatality rate, only second to that of adolescent drivers. Older adult drivers injured in motor vehicle accidents, in turn, are more likely to die as a result than younger drivers. Men, when compared with women, have higher rates for death and injuries from motor vehicle accidents.

There certainly is "life after driving," but the loss of independence is often considered one of the most significant losses resulting from giving up driving, particularly in cases of older adults with considerable disposable income that can be spent on entertainment and dining out (Kim & Richardson, 2006). Cessation of driving may lead to older adult reduction in socialization and fewer out-of-home activities (AGS Foundation for Health in Aging, 2006). Bauer, Rottunda, and Adler's (2003) study of older women and driving cessation, however, found that adaptation was easiest for older women who planned cessation voluntarily. Reliance on others for transportation had the benefit of increasing social contact and reducing loneliness.

Older adults and automobile driving are subjects that make the national news every few years or so. This national attention invariably focuses on an automobile accident that involves older adults as drivers and results in fatal casualties. The headlines invariably stress the question of whether older adults should be allowed to drive because of what their age and potential impairments present to public safety. The discussions that follow usually get quite heated about individual rights versus public safety. Age-related medical or health conditions are often cited as a major cause of this age group being considered a safety risk on the nation's roads (Odenheimer, 2006). Tuokko, Rhodes, and Dean (2007) found that health-related symptoms such as those relating to the spine and lower back stood out in influencing decisions to relinquish driving.

A number of health promotion programs have been advanced in the past decade and no doubt will increase in frequency in the next decade as the numbers of baby boomers enter retirement age (Classen et al., 2006; Windsor & Anstey, 2006). Programs stressing self-regulation and involvement of key actors in an older adult's social network have shown prominence (Rudman, Friedland, & Chipman, 2006). Physicians and nurse practitioners have been targeted by some programs because of their contact and importance in an older adult's life (Carr, Duchek, Meuser, & Morris, 2006; Johnson, 2000; Odenheimer, 2006). Physicians can assist families through provision of information and clarifying state regulations. Further, some state departments of motor vehicles mandate that physicians report specific medication conditions that can severely impair driving. Nurse practitioners, too, have been enlisted in helping older adult drivers in cases where they have forfeited their driver's license, and helping them cope with this loss.

Preretirement programs that help older adults not only transition to life after work but also to a life less reliant on driving have also shown prominence (Adler & Rottunda, 2006). Foley, Heimovitz, Guralnik, and Brock (2002), however, stress the need for health promotion programs to take gender into account. The authors found that women require more years of support for transportation alternatives than their male counterparts because of increased life expectancy.

Driving in this society serves both practical and symbolic values (Freeman, Gange, Munoz, & West, 2006). The freedom and independence associated with driving automobiles is one that is deeply ingrained in the national fabric, and as a result presents a unique set of challenges for health promotion programs. Issues related to individual rights versus the rights of the general public often strike at the heart of the tension related to giving up one's drivers license. Automatically terminating an individual's drivers license based upon age, however, opens the door to other groups losing their rights to drive.

SUBSTANCE ABUSE

Substance use and abuse is a topic that is usually reserved to youth and young adults but rarely raised when discussing older adults (Substance Abuse and Mental Health Services Administration [SAMHSA], 2002). In 2002, 66,500 adults aged fifty-five or older were admitted to substance abuse treatment programs, or 107 per 100,000, which is lower than the rate of 801 per 100,000 for those under the age of fifty-five (SAMHSA, 2006a). The number of admissions represents a 32 percent increase from 1995. Alcohol was the primary drug of abuse with 77.5 percent of those admitted. In 2003, approximately 12 percent of older adults engaged in alcohol binge drinking and 3.2 reported heavy alcohol consumption (SAMHSA, 2006a).

When the subject of substance abuse is raised pertaining to this age group, it usually focuses on abuse of prescription drugs. Abuse of prescription drugs is a major area of concern in programs serving older adults (Torres, 2004). The high rate of abuse and misuse of prescription medications should not come as a great surprise since an average older adult takes 5.3 prescription medications per day; older adults on average use psychotropic drugs two to three times more than younger age groups and also have a higher probability of misusing these medications (Shibusawa, 2006).

Older adult alcohol and drug abuse and misuse is considered one of the fastest growing public health problems in the nation (Shibusawa, 2006). As noted in chapter 2, older adults who have substance abuse problems will increasingly tax current service delivery systems and require specialized programs and settings that take into consideration their age and life experiences (Gross, 2008a). Older adult males are four times more likely than females to abuse alcohol, with African-American and Latino males having even higher rates than white non-Latino males; Latina older adults, in turn, have lower rates than white non-Latinas and African Americans (Shibusawa, 2002). There are estimates that the number of substance-abusing older adults aged fifty years or older will double in size from 2.5 million in 1999 to 5 million in the year 2020 (Gfroerer, Penne, Pemberton, & Folsom, 2003).

Morley (2003, p. M2) comments on an important different dimension to this phenomenon: "It is now well established that older persons often receive excessive numbers of drugs that are often responsible for a variety of negative effects. . . . Nancy Reagan's 'Just say no to drugs' campaign may have produced more results if it had been aimed at seniors instead of teenagers!" Thus, the abuse of prescription drugs is multifaceted and must not be viewed solely from an older adult's perspective, with the medical and pharmaceutical establishment bearing some significant part of the blame.

Prescription medication and alcohol misuse affects up to 17 percent of Americans over the age of sixty-five; older adults use 30 percent of all prescription drugs, yet represent approximately 13 percent of the total population in this country (Sullivan, Lynch, Artesani, & Seed, 2007). As a result, older adults are not immune to substance abuse problems (Barry, Oslin, & Blow, 2001, p. 2): "Despite significant advances over the past two decades in understanding of the aging process with its attendant health problems, little attention has been paid to the intersection where gerontology, or geriatrics, and alcohol studies meet." There are indications that alcohol consumption continues with aging at a higher level than in previous older cohorts (Korper & Raskin, 2007). This problem has not escaped total attention in the field, as evidenced by at least two books written on this topic (Barry et al., 2001; Gurnack, 1999) in the past decade.

Hatchett (1999) studied alcohol misuse among older (aged fifty-five to eighty-nine) African-American women and found the condition to be under-reported and undertreated. Satre and Arean (2005), in their study of the effects of gender, ethnicity, and medical illness on drinking cessation in older primary care patients, found that key demographic factors such as gender wield significant influence. This is particularly relevant in older women with physical illnesses. Kirchner and colleagues (2007) studied alcohol consumption among older adults in primary care and found that heavy drinking was associated with depression and anxiety and less social support.

Excessive drinking of alcohol, for example, can increase health risks related to liver disease, peptic ulcers, hypertension, heart disease, and stroke among older adults (Blow et al., 2000). Andrews (in press) addresses substance abuse among older Latino adults and predicts an increase in alcohol and drug abuse in this population group as Latinos grow in numbers among older adults in the country. However, when addressing older adults of color with very distinctive cultural belief systems that are very different from prevailing beliefs, such as the use of folk medicine and how these beliefs and medicines interact with conventional medicines, prescription use takes on added significance, such as in the case of older adult Latinos (Delgado, 2007). Very little formal information is known about the interactions of folk medicines and prescriptions.

Public and professional perceptions of substance abuse as being a problem for the young and early adults but not one for older adults probably remains the biggest challenge for the field of health promotion (Torres, 2004, p. 1): "Researchers are only beginning to realize the pervasiveness of substance abuse disorders among people aged sixty and older. Until recently, alcohol and prescription drug misuse—which affects as many as 17 percent of older adults—was not discussed in either dependency/ addiction or gerontological literature." Consequently, it becomes a challenge for the public and professionals to think about older adults as possibly being at risk for misusing or abusing alcohol and other drugs, and not just prescription drugs.

Djousse, Biggs, Mukamal, and Siscovick (2007), in a study of alcohol consumption and type-2 diabetes among older adults, found that light to moderate drinking was associated with a lower incidence of diabetes, regardless of the type of alcohol beverage consumed. Resnick's (2003c) findings from a study of alcohol use among older adults in a continuing care retirement community stress the need for health promotion initiatives to be individualized to take into account the benefits and risks to alcohol use. The complexity of the subject necessitates an individualized, although more time-consuming, approach toward health promotion interventions.

The need for new data sources specifically focused on older adults and substance abuse will gain prominence as the baby boomer generation continues to enter retirement age (Korper & Raskin, 2007). Health promotion providers, in turn, must be able and willing to engage in a campaign to uplift this age group for funding and targeted interventions. This will put older adults in competition for funds that have historically been considered the exclusive domain of youth and young adults. Not surprisingly, changing attitudes will present a far greater challenge than developing new models for prevention and treatment of substance abuse among older adults.

Smoking

Tobacco and its various manifestations, but particularly cigarettes, bring a host of health-related problems for all age groups and not just older adults (Eisner et al., 2000; Schiller & Ni, 2006). However, in the case of older adults who have a long history of smoking, it brings serious health consequences and challenges for the reduction or stopping of smoking. It seems like the smoking cessation field has focused on youth and young adults and has largely ignored older adults. Smoking among low-income/low-wealth older adults brings a financial dimension that is generally overlooked in the literature. The cost of purchasing cigarettes takes on added significance in situations where older adults must choose between purchasing cigarettes and purchasing their prescriptions and healthy foods.

It is estimated that in 2003 there were 13.7 million persons aged fifty or older who smoked cigarettes (SAMHSA, 2006b). In the early 2000s, there were over 430,000 smoking-related deaths annually in the United States; of these deaths, approximately 94 percent involved individuals over the age of fifty years, with 70 percent of these deaths involving persons sixty-five years or older (Center for Social Gerontology, 2001). Cancer, heart disease, and stroke represent three of the major causes of death. However, deaths resulting from tobacco-related fires, which are generally overlooked in discussions of tobacco-related casualties, accounted for almost 440 deaths of persons over the age of sixty-five years in 1995 (Center for Social Gerontology, 2001).

Roff and colleagues (2005), however, in a study focused on religiosity, smoking, exercise, and obesity among Southern, community-dwelling older adults, found no association between religiosity and the likelihood of being obese. Like other researchers noted in this book, they recommend faith communities as resources for delivering health promotion to older adults. These institutions enjoy the trust of the communities they serve and have long and often distinguished histories of serving these communities' physical, social, and psychological needs, as well as their spiritual needs.

It is rare to see a public service announcement that targets smoking among older adults. Like substance abuse, prevention and early intervention in smoking cessations have been seen as the province of the young. However, as noted earlier in this section, older adults and smoking is quite complex a subject (Elena, Chen, Kim, & Abdulrahim, 2002). Harm reduction strategies, particularly those involving innovative approaches that incorporate less hazardous tobacco products, are finding their way into health promotion programs (Meier & Shelley, 2006). Resnick (2001a), in summarizing the literature on smoking and the old-old age group, raises the importance of harm reduction, in this case reducing nicotine intake rather than cessation, because of the unlikelihood of a goal of stopping smoking being agreed to by older adults with long histories of smoking.

O'Connell (2001) notes that older smokers generally have a much more difficult time quitting smoking than their younger counterparts, primarily as the result of a longer addiction period to nicotine. Beliefs that it is too late to quit (health damages have already occurred) combine with fears of consequences resulting from withdrawal, making health promotion cessation programs targeting older adults challenging. Nevertheless, the lowering of smoking rates still results in significant numbers of lives being saved, healthier lives, and reduction in health costs for the nation. Arriving at health promotion goals regarding older adult smoking will prove challenging for the field because of the tension between individual rights and health-compromising behaviors. Hard reduction goals, as a result, may be very attractive as a means of addressing the health consequences of smoking while maintaining their rights to smoke.

Gambling

Gambling and older adult health and health promotion seems out of place for most readers. Gambling, after all, is a form of entertainment or leisure that is usually not associated with most forms of social intervention, including health promotion. Nevertheless, gambling becomes a health concern when it interferes with older adults having necessary funds to purchase medications, affects consumption of healthy foods because of costs, interferes with physical activities, and becomes an addiction.

Petry (2002) found that older adult women who could be classified as pathological gamblers did not start gambling until after an average age of fifty-five years, while their male counterparts reported a lifelong history of gambling. Further, older adults constitute a small percentage of those in treatment for gambling. Pietrzak, Mollins, Ladd, Kerins, and Petry (2005) found that older adults with a gambling problem experienced increased severity of health and psychosocial problems when compared with older adults with no or infrequent gambling. Health promotion initiatives related to gambling, as a result, can be expected to increase in frequency in the near future. However, like their smoking counterparts, those favoring restraint will no doubt clash with those favoring restricting gambling.

Legalized gambling is a big business in this country with gross estimates of $50 billion annually being spent on this activity, and with approximately two-thirds of the country's adult population having participated in some form of gambling in the past year (Desai, Maciejewski, Dausey, Caldarone, & Potenza, 2004). The growth of the gambling industry has been sizable over the past several decades, and this is reflected in lifetime gambling participation increases in older adult participation from 35 percent in 1975 to 80 percent in 1998 (Desai et al., 2004). Older adults represent a significant portion of the nation's gambling population, even for those in residential and assisted-living facilities. One study, for example, found that over 6,000 older adults indicated that gambling was one of the most significant social activities that they participated in, with 23 percent attending in-house bingo games at least four times per week (Potenza, Kosten, & Rounsaville, 2001).

Patsdaughter, Christensen, Kelley, Masters, and Ndiwane (2002) report on a study of gambling behaviors of African-American older adults and perceived effects on health. Zaranek and Chapleski (2005) used activity theory to guide their study of urban older adults and gambling and found that gambling, although not a "favorite" activity, is part of a constellation of activities. Preston, Shapiro, and Keene (2007) studied successful aging and gambling among older adults who moved to Las Vegas, Nevada, and found that those older adults who have integrated gambling as part of their recreational outlets are four times more likely to develop a gambling addiction than those who do not. Further, the likelihood of developing a gambling problem increases when video poker is the primary gambling activity.

Gambling, like the other low-profile health needs identified in this chapter, suffers from a lack of recognition or awareness in public and professional arenas as to its impact on the health of older adults. Gambling, too, covers a wide range of activities, from bingo night in local houses of worship and residential settings, to other venues such as casinos, state-sponsored lotteries, and racetracks, for example. Consequently, the importance of targeting health promotion interventions to specific settings must be emphasized, along with specific gambling activities. Like smoking, individual rights will take center stage in the development of health promotion initiatives and the importance of creating positive alternatives to gambling in order to engage older adults.

Violence

The subject of violence is not only complex but also heavily politically charged in this society, regardless of the age group being discussed. There are numerous perspectives that older adult health promotion can take on violence. Exposure to violence brings with it health consequences because of the fear it elicits, and the restrictions that older adults face in socially navigating their community. Gray and Acierno (2002) have found underreporting of older adult trauma victims as well as underdiagnosis by clinicians, masking the consequences of criminal acts against this population group.

The demographic increase in older adults brings with it an increase in those who are subject to abuse, neglect, exploitation, self-neglect, and victims of violent acts (Tomita, 2006). Being the direct subject of violent acts such as street crime elicits a different response from that of elder abuse by family members (Tatara, 1999). Nevertheless, it is impossible to discuss urban living without also noting the potential of urban violence on a population age group that is widely acknowledged to be vulnerable to crime because of physical characteristics, such as lack of fast mobility or physical strength to ward off physical attacks. Cases involving older adults who have been violently attacked often make national news.

There is little dispute professionally and publicly that older adults are susceptible to various forms of violent crime, both outside and within their families. Tomita (2006), for example, identified eight forms of older adult maltreatment and neglect that necessitate different health promotion approaches:

1. physical abuse
2. sexual abuse
3. emotional or psychological abuse
4. financial abuse
5. identity theft
6. undue influence
7. neglect
8. self-neglect

The complexities associated with each of these eight forms of harm necessitates that health promotion assess the context and circumstances that lead to these actions. A one-size-fits-all approach will prove unsuccessful in preventing or minimizing the consequences of violence against older adults.

Injuries and violence among older adults are considered a major cause of disability and death (Stevens et. al., 1999). Chu and Kraus (2004), for example, found that older adults have a higher risk of death resulting from assaults by younger perpetrators. D'Augelli and Grossman (2001), in turn, studied lifetime victimization of sexual minorities sixty years or age or older and found very high rates because of sexual orientation, making this subgroup that much more vulnerable to verbal and physical victimization.

Older adult health promotion specifically focused on violence is still in its infancy, although its importance and prominence will grow as the field starts to grapple with the extreme consequences to health as a result of violence or the threat of violence. Special attention must be placed on the social characteristics that make older adults vulnerable to various forms of physical and psychological violence. Jasinski and Dietz (2003), for example, argue that there are limited data on the extent of older adult physical abuse by spouse or partners. Bonomi and colleagues' (2007) study of intimate partner violence in older women sixty-five years or older found that high lifetime partner violence among older women has long-term adverse health consequences, resulting in a need for specialized efforts to reach these women. Violence against older adults is a public health concern that must find its way into any health promotion initiative targeting older adults in general, and specifically older adults of color residing in the nation's urban areas.

SPECIAL POPULATION GROUPS

The use of the label "special population groups" is arguably arbitrary, yet it captures a particular social situation that often portrays neglect, or fear of society, for a particular demographic group. When the label is applied to an age group and health, as in the case of this book, it captures a social situation whereby a group has suffered disproportionate harm that has caused health conditions to be overlooked or poorly addressed by the health field. The three groups covered in this final section are certainly not monolithic, and it is possible to have an accumulation of factors such as older adults of color who are gay or lesbian and imprisoned, for example. Endless combinations of factors are not just possible but likely, and result in poor health status. When these vulnerabilities are placed within a lifespan context, the "specialness" of their circumstances takes on added significance for older adult health promotion initiatives.

Lesbian, Gay, Bisexual, and Transgender (LGBT) Health Needs

Social context plays such an influential role in how health gets defined and in help-seeking patterns, and this is so much the case when discussing older adults who are LGBT. The role and importance of urban areas in the life of the LGBT community, particularly those who are older adults with long histories of living in cities, is unmistakable (Finkelstein & Netherland, 2005). Cities have historically been places of refuge for sexual minority groups, and continue to be so even today. Health promotion targeting these individuals, as a result, has a prominent place in urban-based health promotion.

Donahue and McDonald (2005) conclude that relatively little empirical knowledge can be found about older adults who are gay and lesbian, and the same can be said about those who are bisexual and transgendered. The health needs of older adults cannot be viewed through a narrow lens with a focus on heterosexual older adults (Mail & Safford, 2003; Shankle, Maxwell, Katzman, & Landers, 2003). The inclusion of a population group that represents an alternative view of gender, sexual identity, and sexual orientation, is a worthy and important subject to be included in this book. However, LGBT older adults can be found in all communities, including communities of color, and they, too, face health care challenges in having their health care needs met in a culturally competent manner that affirms their identity and beliefs!

Chapin, Nelson-Becker, Gordon, and Terrebonne (2002), in a rare article specifically devoted to this special population group, note that the group will number about 4 million by 2030. One 2007 estimate has the gay, lesbian, and bisexual fifty-five years and older population numbering 2.4 million, with same-sex couples numbering 416,000 (Gross, 2007). Butler (2006) estimates that the nation's gay, lesbian, and bisexual population numbers between 1 million and 2.8 million, with a projected increase to between 2 and 6 million by the year 2030. Transgendered persons are estimated to number about 3 percent of all older adults. Not surprisingly, estimates of LGBT populations are arduous to arrive at due to significant bias in national population surveys, as reflected by the wide range of estimates presented above (Zodikoff, 2006).

Davies (2001), in examining the topic of sexuality and older adults, raises what is probably the greatest challenge facing the field when discussing homosexual and lesbian health promotion:

> If there are barriers to heterosexual contact in older people there are even greater barriers to homosexual and lesbian relationships. It is relatively recently that homosexual relationships have been made legal and for many people they are still not acceptable, particularly to older people who grew up when homosexuality was a criminal offense. Many older women form close loving relationships with other women yet never transfer their feelings into any form of physical expression. Overcoming these barriers should be a way of providing affectionate touch or someone to share a bed (p. 89).

A front-page *New York Times* article titled "Aging and Gay, and Facing Prejudice in Twilight" (Gross, 2007) makes aging and LGBT older adults a public concern and not just for academics. This article raises the stigma that these older adults face and the isolation and pain that result when they "come out" in residential settings where the majority of the residents are heterosexual.

LGBT older adults, due to social circumstances regarding long histories of bias and discrimination, require health promotion initiatives that take into account the unique place they occupy in the older adult population (Davis, 2006). California is currently the only state in the nation with a law that acknowledges that older adult gays have special needs that necessitate group-specific targeting (Gross, 2007). In cases where they also happen to be of color, their health status is further compromised, and there is a need for concerted attention from the field. These special initiatives will prove controversial, and this is to be expected. However, the alternative—to continue to ignore the health needs of this population group—represents an even more distressing stance for the field. The emergence of older adult social clubs that are LGBT-specific represents an effort to introduce an atmosphere for older adults to enjoy social contacts and reduce isolation, a key dimension in any LGBT health promotion initiative (Gross, 2007).

Homelessness

It is impossible to discuss older adult health promotion within an urban context and not recognize older adults who are homeless, nationally and internationally (Bephage, 2006; Crane et al., 2005; Health Research Resources and Services Administration, 2003; Hahn, Kushel, Bangsberg, Riley, & Moss, 2006; Lee, Hanlon, & Ben-David, 2005). Although homelessness is not a phenomenon unique to cities, its manifestation in urban areas brings forth vivid visual images that rural homelessness simply does not. Concentrations of homeless older adults in certain public sectors of cities such as parks, outside of major buildings, and under major thoroughfares, are quite common. Homeless older adults, like their older adult counterparts who are not homeless, can be quite diverse in composition (Bottomley, Bissonette, & Snekvik, 2001; Brucker, 2001; Crane & Warnes, 2001; Downes & Channer, 2001). Like their incarcerated counterparts, however, fifty years is considered the beginning of older age (Cohen, Sokovsky, & Crane, 2001).

It is estimated that older adults fifty years or older constitute anywhere between 14.8 and 28.0 percent of the homeless population in the United States, but those estimates are quite dated (Garibaldi, Conde-Martel, & O'Toole, 2005). O'Connell (2005) concluded that a homeless person is three to four times more likely to die than the general population. Illnesses can be spread quite easily among the homeless, and these can be made more lethal by exposure to the elements.

Issues related to victimization of older adults who are homeless (Dietz & Wright, 2005a,b), for example, place these individuals at increased risk for violence. The prevalence of psychiatric illnesses (Bartles, 2003; Nabonezny & Ojeda, 2005; Washington, 2005) and HIV (Emlet & Poindexter, 2004; Hwang et al., 2001) also further compound the lives of older adults who are homeless. Garibaldi and colleagues (2005) found in their study of homelessness in Pittsburgh and Philadelphia that older homeless persons were 3.6 times more likely to report medical conditions, 2.8 times more likely not to have some form of health insurance, and 2.4 times more likely to be dependent on heroin than their counterparts under the age of fifty years old. Kessell, Bhatia, Bamberger, and Kushel (2006), too, found homeless older adults to have great health needs. In one San Francisco study, homeless older adults had an asthma rate twice what it would normally be expected to be (White, Tulsky, Dawson, Zolopa, & Moss, 1997).

Quine, Kendig, Russell, and Touchard (2004), in a study of homeless older men in Australia, identified a range of health promotion goals and service strategies that take into account the unique social circumstances these men faced trying to survive in the streets. The setting(s) where health promotion initiatives transpire must embrace innovation and a willingness to venture into arenas that the field may be unaccustomed to in order to be effective. Health promotion in city parks, alleys, and other places where the homeless congregate, including day shelters, must be part of any serious health promotion initiative.

Prison Health Promotion

The reader may be initially surprised by the possibility of health promotion in prisons, let alone having it target older adult inmates. The image of older adults who are inmates is probably not first and foremost in the nation's mind when discussing incarcerated inmates. As noted in chapter 1, older adulthood is generally defined as being fifty years and older for the nation's inmates. However, some researchers have started to recommend that the age be lowered to forty-five years to better represent the physical and emotional state of these inmates (Yorston & Taylor, 2006).

As a result of a number of significant forces that have been operating in this country, the nation's prison inmates are slowly undergoing transformation to the point that older adults are becoming an increasingly larger portion of the prison population. Between 1990 and 2001, for example, their numbers increased from 4 percent of the prison population to 8.2 percent, more than doubling in size (Yorston & Taylor, 2006). Further, the period from 2000 to 2005, for example, witnessed an increase of 33 percent in the number of inmates age fifty-five and older in the nation's prisons, which is faster than the 9 percent growth overall (Associated Press, 2007). This transformation of prison inmates, however, is not restricted to the United States.

The United Kingdom's prisons, too, are experiencing a fast growth in the older adult (sixty years and older) inmate population, with this age group being the fastest growing sector of the inmate population ("Prison's ageing population," 2006). This group is not too dissimilar from its U.S. counterparts, with 85 percent having at least one major illness and 83 percent reporting at least one chronic illness or disability ("Prison's ageing population," 2006).

Not unexpectedly, morbidity and mortality are very high among older adult inmates (Linder & Meyers, 2007). Aday (2006, p. 234) summarizes a large number of health studies on older adults in prisons: "On average, these studies found a significant incidence of chronic illness for ailments such as arthritis (41 percent), heart disease (26 percent), menopause problems (33 percent), prostate problems (18 percent), emphysema (20 percent), stomach disorders (17 percent), diabetes (12 percent), cancer (6 percent), and stroke (8 percent)." Older adult prisoners on average have three or more chronic illnesses and take even more medications.

Health promotion in correctional settings such as prison is a concept that is almost thirty years old and originally appeared in the professional literature in the middle 1980s (E. M. Gallagher & Beecher, 1987). Nevertheless, the widespread use of this intervention has not occurred, even though prisons and jails are places where health promotion can make a dramatic difference in the health of inmates. When older adult health promotion efforts are launched within prisons, prisoner rights and ethical dilemmas often emerge due to the context of these total institutions (Yorston & Taylor, 2006).

Loeb, Steffensmeier, and Lawrence (2008) found that there were no significant differences between older adult men who were incarcerated and those in the community, when examining self-efficacy for health management or health status. There were, however, significant differences in participation in health promotion programs, and this may be the result of a lack of availability or awareness of such programs. Loeb and Steffensmeier (2006), in an extremely rare article on older male prisoners and health promotion, stress the need for the field to pay closer attention to this special population group and develop interventions that enhance health knowledge and self-efficacy within prisons. Kuhlmann and Ruddell (2005) address older adults in county jails and advocate for health promotion initiatives for this age group, but they acknowledge that jails tend to be smaller than prisons and inmates stay for shorter sentences, creating challenges beyond those normally encountered in prisons. Correctional context, as a result, necessitates that any health promotion efforts be tailored to local circumstances.

There certainly is a major difference between individuals who are of ill health and population groups that are ill. Development of an understanding of illness and disease that results from society's actions or inactions is much more than semantics. Actions needed to address the causes of these illnesses must ultimately be a prominent part of any urban-focused health promotion strategy that hopes to make a significant impact on the health of marginalized older adults.

Older adults, particularly those from certain low-income/low-wealth, ethnic, and racial backgrounds, face a wide range of well-recognized and unrecognized illnesses and diseases in this society, making them a group worthy of special attention from the field of health promotion. This chapter stands as a testament to the health needs of this population group and highlights the devastating consequences that result from long histories of being exposed to toxic environments and lacking access to quality health care (Szczepura, 2005). These health needs, however, rarely stand alone and very often are found in combinations of various types. Comorbidity, as a result, further complicates the delivery of health services, including health promotion.

Some of the health needs addressed in this chapter probably did not represent any surprise to the reader, while others certainly did. Clearly, there are other health needs that will emerge in the near future that will come as a surprise to the reader as well as myself. In many ways, the field of health promotion is entering uncharted waters pertaining to urban older adults of color. As a consequence, the field must be prepared and willing to entertain conditions that on initial observation may not be considered "health" related but upon closer observation do fall within this category, particularly when placed within a socioecological context.

The older adult health promotion field will only continue to grow in the next few decades as the numbers of older adults continue to increase and the oldest of the old also increases. The field must become, as a result, strategic in better addressing a wide range of health concerns, particularly for special population groups that have suffered from even greater neglect in the past. The creation of new methods for gathering and interpreting data will be needed to inform health promotion efforts.

SECTION 2:
HEALTH PROMOTION
THEORY AND PRACTICE

"Transforming the aging of America will require new ideas and new policies—and a new constituency for change—it will especially require new institutions. If we can devise creative new roles and opportunities at the community level, there is much reason to believe that people will respond. . . . [There] is a deep hunger on the part of older Americans to live lives that matter, to use their experience and knowledge in important ways, and to continue learning and growing in the process."

(Freedman, 1999, p. 23)

5

~~

Health Promotion Field

"Indeed, aging is conceptualized as a problem and the paradigm of midlife decline is well documented and reinforced daily through advertisements as well as in textbooks used to educate the next generation of professionals. . . . The paradigm of midlife decline must be replaced with one that creates expectation of continued growth and development through all stages of life."

(Chapin & Cox, 2001, p. 168)

Health promotion, as the reader will see in this chapter, is a highly contextualized intervention strategy that often relies upon multiple theories and not only seeks to empower older adults, but also seeks to alter environmental circumstances that are detrimental to their healthy living and that of their community. This perspective toward health promotion is predicated on "unconventional" borders and settings, and its strategies can cover a wide spectrum, which will often involve social advocacy and social action (Brown, 2007; Delgado & Staples, 2008; Kreuter, 2005; Quiroz-Martinez, Wu, & Zimmerman, 2005). Stokols (2000), as a result, stresses the need for the field to broaden its reach to include strategies that combine behavioral, organizational, environmental, regulatory, and political initiatives as a means of more effectively fulfilling its mission to society. This chapter is conceptualized in this tradition.

Health is no longer viewed as a physical state of being that is absent of diseases and illnesses. This definition is too static and does not do justice to the dynamic and richness of a concept. Further, it effectively looks at health outside of any social context such as culture and spirituality, to list but two key factors. Galea and Vlahov (2005), for example, stress the importance of cross-national research to develop greater knowledge about the key aspects of cities and how urbanization influences population health across groups as a means of grounding health promotion within a specific urban social context.

HEALTH AND HEALTH PROMOTION ON
A NATIONAL AND INTERNATIONAL STAGE

In 2005, the World Health Organization established the Commission on the Social Determinants of Health with a final report to be issued in May 2008, representing an important theoretical and political move toward validating the contextualization of health in a broader social arena. Numerous scholars have moved this area forward toward this goal with progressive thinking. Rabiner (2005), for example, stresses the importance of health promotion involvement consisting of a multidimensional conceptual understanding of older adults within a social context. A social context of health such as urban versus rural, for example, brings with it an emphasis on social determinants. Further, as Burton and Whitfield (2003) argue based on their study of urban low-income families and comorbidity, there is a high level of familial comorbidity, necessitating health promotion strategies that contextualize older adult health within a familial, as well as community, context as a means of increasing its reach and potential impact.

Roberta and Lee (2002), in turn, stress the need to understand the complexity between race, individual socioeconomic status, and the social environment in order to better understand racial differences in health among older adults. The measurement of socioeconomic status of older adults, a critical element in any effort to better ascertain health inequities in this group, is not without controversy. Grundy and Holt (2001), for example, have concluded that using educational attainment or social class paired with a deprivation indicator holds the greatest promise for the field to understand health inequities. Aneshensel and colleagues (2007) make similar observations and recommendations, in this case involving depressive symptoms among older adults. Social context, as a result, is critical to making older adult health promotion relevant (Green, Lewis, Wang, Pearson, & Rivers, 2004).

In addition, health promotion interventions must be sufficiently flexible in design to take into account a wide range of local circumstances (Galloway, 2003). Tannahill (1985), almost a quarter of a century ago, conceptualized health promotion as consisting of three overlapping spheres that are still prevalent today: health education, disease prevention, and health protection. Bunton and Macdonald (2002) observe that health promotion's rapid rise during the last two decades of the twentieth century brought with it "ferment" and "debate," leading to the title of the "new public health." The new public health title is meant to separate out present-day public health initiatives from those of previous decades, and it sets the tone for the need for innovative thinking that is both bold and participatory in outlook.

Cookie-cutter health promotion interventions will not move the field forward in a responsible way in addressing the needs of any age group, let alone older adults (Delgado & Zhou, 2008)! Loeb (2006), for example, in a qualitative (focus groups) study of African-American older adults with chronic health conditions and their coping strategies, identified seven primary strategies:

1. dealing with it
2. exercising
3. seeking information
4. relying on God
5. changing dietary practices
6. self-monitoring
7. self-efficacy

The interplay of all or a combination of some of these strategies must be taken into account in any design of older adult health promotion. Each of these strategies brings with it a set of values, beliefs, or attitudes that cannot be simply ignored in any health promotion effort.

Young and Hayes (2002), in their edited book titled *Transforming Health Promotion Practice: Concepts, Issues, and Applications,* put forth a client/consumer-centered model of health promotion that is holistic in character and very much in line with the thrust of the older adult-led health promotion advanced in this book. These authors, however, raise a series of challenges that the field must successfully navigate through in order to achieve its potential. Freudenberg (2007), in turn, comments on the current state of health promotion and issues a series of challenges for the field:

> Health promotion provides a powerful tool for improving health in the 21st century, but researchers and practitioners have yet to achieve consensus on its scope. Globalization, urbanization, an aging population, and rising rates of chronic diseases are creating new challenges throughout the world. How can health professionals respond to these changing challenges? What are the relevant paradigms for promoting health today? How can universities help move health promotion into a new era? (p. 1).

The International Union for Health Promotion and Education, with important support from the Canadian Consortium for Health Promotion Research and the Public Health Agency of Canada, have promulgated action recommendations that will shape how health promotion is conceptualized on an international scale in the immediate future ("Shaping the future," 2008).

Buchanan (2000), in his book on health promotion, provides a scathing critique of health promotion that reinforces many of the key arguments made in this book:

> Thinking in the field of health promotion is currently framed by the scientific terminology of morbidity and mortality rates, risk factors, randomized control trials, independent and dependent variables, null hypothesis, cost-benefit analyses, and effective behavior change techniques. This book recommends a new direction marked by the concepts of well-being, integrity, values, autonomy, responsibility, civility, caring, and solidarity (p. 3).

Altman and Sevick (2002, p. 137), in their review of Buchanan's book, agree with much of what the author advocates. However, they go on to note the particular significance of the tension between public policy and individual autonomy: "Although Buchanan presents his thesis as an 'ethic' for health promotion, he fails to determine how much autonomy we are willing to trade in order to achieve fairness or better health for our citizens. . . . We also believe that science can help seed dialogue about these issues." The "harshness" of some of the critiques levied at health promotion is probably the result of very high expectations for this method; these critiques are meant to improve the profession rather than get interpreted as "demeaning" the profession (Duncan, 2004).

This chapter seeks to ground the reader in the evolution, goals, qualities, definition of health, theories, common strategies, and challenges, as well as rewards found in this field of practice. There is a tremendous imbalance between social investments in medical care when compared to prevention, and McGinnis, Williams-Russo, and Knickman (2002) make a case for more active policy attention to health promotion and older adults as a means of shifting this imbalance in focus.

The reader will quickly discover the complexities and rewards of delivering health promotion in general, and particularly when addressing older adults (Hartman-Stein & Potkanowicz, 2003; Minkler, Schauffler, & Clements-Nolle, 1999; Richardson, 2006). One researcher noted the importance of social context in the field of health promotion with older adults within an urban context (News-Medical.Net, 2005): "So much of our health-promotion activities have focused on the person and the individual characteristics that make it easier to be healthy. . . . But you can only go so far talking about personal characteristics; you need to better understand the context in which people live so that you can have more of an impact on their health behaviors." This chapter has, as a result, a primary goal contextualizing health promotion in a manner that embraces social causes of illness and diseases, and embraces a social and economic justice perspective as a means of better understanding and addressing the social inequalities that result in health disparities in the nation's cities. This perspective, value, or bias, if you wish, must be made explicit for readers to make their own determination of how one author's view is similar or dissimilar from their own views, and incidentally, is very much in line with the current thrust of the field.

EVOLUTION OF HEALTH PROMOTION

There are probably countless numbers of interpretations for the birth and evolution of the health promotion field (Berridge, 2004). Minkler (2000), however, provides a concise summary of the dominant views of health promotion in the United States and traces it back to the 1970s and a profound disillusionment with medicine, efforts to curtail costs, and the prevailing movement toward self-help and individual control over one's own health. The field of health promotion is over twenty-five years old, complex, and with no "single driver" responsible for its evolution and widespread acceptance (Catford, 2004).

The Canadian Ministry of Health and Welfare issued a report (Lalonde Report) in 1974 titled *A New Perspective on the Health of Canadians*, and this is widely acknowledged as the first introduction of the concept of health promotion (Berridge, 2004; Macdonald & Burton, 2002). However, its international origins have arguably been traced back to a historic World Health Organization (WHO) meeting at Alma Ata (Kazak of the former Soviet Union) in 1978. This meeting resulted in a shifting of power from professional providers to consumers and communities. This shift, in combination with a general dissatisfaction on the part of some health providers concerning an elitist approach toward service delivery, resulted in a conducive context for the emergence of health promotion and the embrace of such concepts and paradigms as capacity enhancement and empowerment (Catford, 2004; Hsueh & Yeh, 2006; Freudenberg, 2004). "Ownership" is often the phrase that is used to symbolize empowerment and the potential for capacity enhancement that results from participation in decision making (Baker, 2001). Tilford (2000) notes that health promotion evolved out of earlier efforts at health education; this evolution has broadened the health promotion scope while managing to keep health education as a vital component.

In 1986, in Ottawa, Canada, the first *International Conference on Health Promotion* was held; it was an historic occasion, and many in the field view this meeting as the "cradle" of health promotion as practiced throughout the world. An encompassing definition of health promotion emerged as a result (Ottawa Charter for Health Promotion, 1986):

> Health promotion is the process of enabling people to increase control over, and to improve, their health. To reach a state of complete physical, mental and social well-being, an individual or group must be able to identify and to realize aspirations, to satisfy needs, and to change or cope with the environment. Health is, therefore, seen as a resource for everyday life, not the objective of living. Health is a positive concept emphasizing social and personal resources, as well as physical capacities. Therefore, health promotion is not just the responsibility of the health sector, but goes beyond healthy life-style to well-being (p. 1).

Collins and Hayes (2007), however, in commemorating the twentieth anniversary of the Ottawa Charter for Health Promotion, note that the continued persistence of health disparities and the conflicting political challenges and ideologically driven resistance still exist. The race toward health promotion goals must be conceptualized as a marathon rather than a sprint in order to better appreciate the difficulties of eliminating health disparities.

On the national front, O'Neill (2002) traces the evolution of health promotion through a series of federal government reports, such as the 1979 surgeon general report *Healthy People: Health Promotion and Disease Prevention*, followed by the 1990s *Healthy People 2000*, and the most current report titled *Healthy People 2010*. Haber (2007, p. 1) also considers the 1979 surgeon general report to be extremely influential in moving the field forward: "Over the years, this report was widely cited by the popular media as well as in professional journals and at health conferences. Many attribute to it a seminal role in fostering health-promoting initiatives throughout the nation." These federal reports have sought to increase the quality and years of healthy life and also sought to eliminate health disparities or inequalities.

The evolution of health promotion since shows no signs of slowing in the early part of the twenty-first century (Acton & Carter, 2006; Allegrante, 2006; Buchanan, 2006). This can be exciting as well as a cause for concern. However, the following are words of warning that must not be ignored (Catford, 2004):

> As we look over the horizon into the next century, the picture is getting bigger and the terrain more hazardous. Although we have much to celebrate concerning the development of health promotion knowledge and practice over the past two decades, we dare not be complacent. . . . Leadership development coupled with a focus on the social determinants of health seem to be key ingredients for the continued growth and well-being of health promotion (p. 4).

Catford (2004) raises important aspects of expansion that cannot be easily ignored if the field of health promotion is to continue to wield tremendous influence in the future.

Some in the field may call for greater use of economics to help continue to fuel the expansion of health promotion in the early part of this century. Whitehead (2006), in a review of the literature on health promotion and nursing, concluded that health promotion continues to be conceptualized as health education and disease-specific prevention, instead of embracing a broader social, economic, political, and ecological perspective. A narrow and apolitical perspective on health promotion involving older adults from marginalized backgrounds may not be viewed as relevant, thereby seriously limiting who participates and the benefits they derive from doing so.

Sindall (2002), in an editorial in the journal *Health Promotion International*, warns that although the field has progressed significantly in the past two decades, it has not made comparable progress in articulating moral and ethical standards. Mittelmark (2008) stresses the need to codify ethics for the field for it to remain true to its mission. As addressed in chapter 8, these standards have taken on greater importance as health promotion has ventured out into new arenas and has embraced a multifaceted agenda to address social determinants of health. This challenge complements the concerns raised by Catford (2004) above and adds a dimension usually not discussed. Further, as the field embraces new population groups such as urban youth of color and older adults of color, for example, critical cultural and social considerations enter into decision making, raising ethical dilemmas and the need for ethical standards and decision making. This is not to say that the field has not been guilty of overlooking important population groups, however.

Rimmer's (1999) observations almost ten years ago about the absence of health promotion efforts focused on people with disabilities are still prevalent today. Drum, Krahn, Culley, and Hammond (2005) raise the need and importance of health promotion addressing the needs of those with disabilities by helping these individuals become "joint managers" of their own health care and engage in healthy behaviors. The authors go on to note that a number of factors, such as economic costs and limited physical mobility, may hamper participation in conventional health promotion programs. Changing demographics will require that the field change to facilitate equitable participation by people with disabilities, particularly those who are older adults (Pandya, 2005).

Charlesworth (2000), in examining disabilities from a caregiving perspective, found mortality rates to be high for older adults who cared for spouses with disabilities. Health promotion programs targeting caregivers of spouses with disabilities are almost nonexistent. The National

Center on Physical Activity and Disability (2004) recommends that more attention be paid to reaching people with disabilities using community-based health promotion. The primary aim of health promotion with people with disabilities is to reduce secondary conditions such as obesity, hypertension, and blood pressure scores, for example, and to facilitate functional independence, provide opportunities for leisure, and enhance overall quality of life. Health promotion that is community based serves to reduce environmental barriers to these goals.

The field of health promotion, too, will continue to expand into new and unchartered waters, such as health promotion and heart failure, prisons, long-term care facilities, gambling, sexually transmitted diseases, and new settings such as beauty parlors, barbershops, community gardens, parks, and health clubs, to cite but a few examples (A. P. Clark et al., 2006; Orsega-Smith, Mowen, Payne, & Godbey, 2004; Pandya, 2005). The move to "Health in All Policies" represents an important attempt to integrate health into all policies addressing economic and social life as a means of tackling health disparities (Kickbusch, McCann, & Sherbon, 2008). Levin and Ashton (2006) embrace a view of health promotion that has its share of advocates. The promotion of health is too important to be relegated to a small sector of society (health promoters) and must engage all sectors of society. Further, health promotion must not corner itself into focusing exclusively on lifestyle changes and thereby engaging in a blaming-the-victim mentality.

Sirianni and Friedland (2001, p. 13) observe that citizen organizing in the health care arena has not risen to its potential to effect significant social change, but the time may be right for this to change: "Innovative democratic and community health approaches that mobilize civic networks and engage citizens in collaborative public work with health professionals and institutions now offer important alternatives to the hegemony of the medical model of acute care for improving the health of populations." Older adult-led health promotion represents one "innovative" approach toward citizenry participation and empowerment (individual as well as community), and brings with it the potential to also engage in citizen organizing to address social justice environmental issues. Community organizing for social change, as a result, is not restricted to younger age groups or social issues that generate outrage on the part of undervalued groups and their communities (Delgado & Staples, 2008).

Health education is often considered a very attractive and popular way of implementing health promotion, but there can be significant differences between health education and promotion. McKenzie and Smeltzer (2001, p. 3) note: "Another term that is closely related to health education, and sometimes incorrectly used in its place, is health promotion. Health promotion is a broader term than health education." There is no denying that there is a strong relationship between these two terms, as evidenced by a book such as *Principles & Foundations of Health Promotion and Education* (Cottrell, Girvan, & McKenzie, 2002) that combines these two areas. Simply stated, health education can stand alone, whereas health promotion can encompass health education as well as a myriad of other strategies.

GOALS AND STRATEGIES OF HEALTH PROMOTION

Health promotion goals can best be thought of as inspirational. Goals that are not inspirational generally fail to capture the attention and excitement of a field. Health promotion and older adults refers to a way of thinking and acting about health and this age group. Like its youth-led health promotion counterpart, for example, health promotion and older adults is not just about achieving a healthy state of being (Delgado & Zhou, 2008). Health promotion is also about challenging conventional thinking and approaches toward health and older adults. This form of health promotion embraces a set of values and strategies that are deeply grounded within a social and economic justice perspective, viewing health from an ecological vantage point, and seeing social change as a viable and essential goal of any strategy involving older adults (Liss, 2000). Older adult psychological well-being is closely tied to housing quality, for example, reinforcing the importance of an ecological perspective on health promotion (Evans, Kantrowitz, & Eshelman, 2002).

The health promotion field, however, conjures up a variety of different definitions and goals (Bunton & Macdonald, 2002):

> To many social and political activists working to combat the social organization of ill health, it was akin to a new social movement, and a rallying point around which to fight for better health. . . . To others health promotion represented a new way of addressing contemporary health and social care policy needs. . . . For yet others, health promotion was an exciting intellectual development that presented new theoretical challenges drawing upon a social, as opposed to bio-medical model of health. The possibilities for empowerment, participation, capacity building, and enhancing social capital were not simply a theoretical, values-driven endeavor, but one that had implications for methodology, research, and professional practice (p. 1).

Thus, the "broadness" of health promotion lends itself to a variety of goals depending upon the perspective of those in this field.

Three key factors have been identified as extremely influential in affecting health in the nation's cities: (1) the physical environment, (2) the social environment, and (3) access to health and social services (Galea & Vlahov, 2005). Each of these factors, in turn, takes on greater significance when applied to older adults who are undervalued because of low-wealth/low-income, race/ethnicity, sexual orientation, and beliefs, thus influencing the goals and strategies of health promotion.

Onge, Rogers, and Denney's (2004) study of obesity within the context of neighborhood, for example, found that racial and socioeconomic composition are positively associated with risk for obesity. Zenk and colleagues (2005), too, raise the deleterious health consequences of racial and class segregation (Detroit) and how the lack of access to supermarkets increases the likelihood of diet-related diseases. Yeh and colleagues (2008), in turn, advocate for health promotion strategies increasing access to fresh fruit and vegetables as a means of helping to fight certain cancers and reduce morbidity and mortality from heart disease and obesity. Thus, health promotion initiatives targeting obesity cannot single out older adults without also taking into account the role of neighborhood. In essence, one's place of residence affects obesity status (Lopez, 2007).

Freudenberg (2007), in reporting on some of the outcomes of the 2006 Meeting of the National Expert Panel on Community Health Promotion, noted that concerns were raised about the limitations of an approach to health promotion that fails to take into account key determinants of lifestyle. Further, conventional approaches that blame the victims and do not address changing policy are doomed to fail. An increase in age is often associated with an increase in certain types of illnesses and diseases, making the case for harm reduction interventions that are specifically targeted to certain health conditions. For example, it is estimated that 60 percent of cancer occurs in people over the age of sixty-five years (Penson, Daniels, & Lynch, 2004). Further, treatment of cancer in this age group is complicated when other illnesses co-occur. Sahay, Ashbury, Roberts, and Rootman (2006), in an extensive review of the literature on nutrition, found a strong relationship between cancer and nutrition, for example.

Hertzman (2004, p. 150), like a number of other scholars, strongly advocates for the use of life-course factors as a means of creating a better understanding of general well-being and physical and chronic diseases among older adults: "Exposure to both beneficial and adverse circumstances over the life-course will vary for each individual and will constitute a unique 'life exposure trajectory' that will manifest itself in different expressions of health and well-being." Moody-Ayers, Lindquist, Sen, and Covinsky (2007), in turn, found that childhood socioeconomic status affects health status through midlife, but the consequences may weaken in late life, offering some degree of hope concerning slowing of the long-term consequences of early lifetime illnesses.

The understanding of the influence of community or neighborhood on health, as a result, has increased in significance this past decade, particularly for health promotion, when examining and addressing health disparities among older adults in low-wealth and low-income circumstances (Mendes, de Leon, & Glass, 2004; Morenoff & Lynch, 2004). This ecological-focused approach has made health promotion as an intervention more attractive to academics and practitioners who embrace empowerment and participatory values and principles for practice. Urban neighborhoods that are severely under-resourced highlight the negative influential determination role of social environment on health (Vlahov et al., 2007).

Nevertheless, the quest to "conquer" the new frontier of community for the field of health promotion brings with it both joys and frustrations associated with the entry into a "new" arena that we are often ill-prepared for (McKnight, 1994):

> The dilemma we face is lack of familiarity with the real community. We have great professional skills in managing and working within our systems, but our skills are much less developed once we leave the system's space and cross over the frontier into the community. Indeed, many professionals are confused and frustrated when they attempt to work in community space, which seems very complex, disoriented, unstructured, and uncontrollable. And many health professionals begin to discover that their powerful tools and techniques seem weaker, less effective, and even inappropriate in the community (p. 24).

Older adult health promotion can also encompass other goals that may not be directly tied to health behaviors and outcomes. Saving funds, for example, may be a goal, particularly in government-sponsored initiatives. Goetzel (2007) concluded that older adult health promotion not only increases their well-being, it can also result in saving the federal government Medicare funds because of increased health benefits resulting from these interventions. Ozminkowski and colleagues (2006) stress the potential of saving medical costs and advocate for the federal government to undertake randomized trials. Health promotion takes on added significance for older adults since it is estimated that 30 cents of every dollar spent on Medicare is devoted to end-of-life care (McCabe-Sellers & Johnston, 2006). However, saving taxpayer money through health promotion is considered to be a misguided use of economics, according to Cohen and Hale (2002, p. 178): "Economics provides the framework for considering how efficiently health promotion achieves its objectives and how health promotion resources can be used most cost-effectively. Economics also provides an analysis of health-promoting behaviours and of the incentives that exist to prevent ill health or to engage in activities that damage health."

The Ottawa Charter of 1986 identifies five primary strategies to promote health and highlights a range of possible approaches to health promotion:

1. build healthy public policy through legislation, fiscal measures, taxation, and organizational change
2. create supportive environments that generate optimal living and working conditions
3. strengthen community actions that empower communities to own and control their own endeavors and destinies
4. develop personal skills that enable people to learn and cope with chronic illness and injuries
5. reorient health services through research, professional education, and training, to create and sustain healthier individuals and communities

The goals often associated with health promotion initiatives can be conceptualized as either "achievable" or what I like to think of as "the impossible dream." The former are realistic. However, critics argue that these goals sell the profession far short of its potential. The latter, in turn, are not achievable but represent the ideals that motivate or inspire us to do better. Critics, however, argue that impossible goals set the field up for guaranteed failure. The reader must ultimately decide which side they subscribe to: those goals that are feasible and most likely to be achieved, or those that serve as a motivator but will not see fruition in our lifetime. Regardless of where we stand, health promotion goals must seek to better the health of all people, and particularly those who are most vulnerable to disease and illness in our society.

HEALTH PROMOTION SETTINGS

There are certainly numerous perspectives on how best to appreciate and understand health promotion settings. Health promotion settings can best be appreciated and understood as an extension of context, or as a specific entity within context. Wenzel (1997) provides a definition of settings that is sufficiently dynamic to accommodate the broad and encompassing aspects of health promotion: "a frame of face-to-face, social interaction among human beings, the meaning of which is socially and culturally shared within the particular group of people being a part of the setting for a certain period of time. That is, this particular meaning of the setting may vary among different social groups at different points in time; it may even be non-existent for other social groups at the same time."

McQueen (2000), among others, states that "settings" are critical to grounding health promotion theory and practice, making it impossible to fully conceptualize health promotion as a field without paying due attention to the role settings play in helping the field carry out its mission. However, health promotion settings, like health promotion itself, have evolved over the past few decades and have slowly encompassed places and spaces that have historically not been associated with health promotion and older adults. Primary settings (Allen, 2001), however, have enjoyed considerable popularity within the field. Nakasato and Carnes (2006), in turn, advocate for greater attention in primary care settings to be paid to health promotion, particularly since these settings are familiar and experience high levels of contact with older adults. Health promotion targeting older adults, nevertheless, can transpire in a variety of settings, formal and informal.

McWilliam and colleagues (1999), for example, see health promotion as playing an important role in helping recently hospital-discharged older adults make a successful transition home, with health promotion transpiring in the home. The authors concluded (McWilliam et al., 1999, pp. 37–38): "Health professionals can proceed to refine person-centered, health-centered, participatory approaches to care. . . . Health care delivery strategies which include care focused on health, as opposed to illness, are clearly warranted, as are efforts to convey more consciously professional attitudes which recognize shared authority on care." Residential settings (Squire, 2001), however, have historically not been the focus of health promotion initiatives, although that is starting to change. This may, in part, be the result of a fundamental and very biased and dated belief that older adult residents could not benefit from health promotion.

Clift and Morrisey (2001) in many ways typify how the field of older adult health promotion has outgrown its conventional boundaries and reached out into new areas of practice:

> As the older population of Western societies continues to grow, and assumes a greater proportion of the total population, so the number of older travelers will increase, with an increasing need for primary health care professionals to provide support and sound practical advice to help people to realize their remaining dreams of travel (p. 142).

Health promotion in this arena, for example, does not have to be restricted to where it can transpire. Airports and other travel arenas such as train and bus stations, for example, can be settings for older adult–targeted health promotion. Just like shopping malls have increased in prominence as places to provide a wide variety of services for older adults and other age groups, travel-related settings, too, can be seen as viable places and spaces for health promotion to be provided.

The emergence of cafes in not-for-profit settings has started to draw older adults in a nonstigmatizing manner and offer a wide variety of activities that are health education focused (Gross, 2008b). Linnan and Ferguson (2007) advocate for the use of beauty salons as health promotion settings for outreach to African-American women. These settings provide easy access within the community and are considered ideal for outreaching to women. Delgado (1999) labeled these types of community settings as "nontraditional" settings, or places in a community where residents can purchase a product or service, or simply congregate, and while doing so receive some form of human service. This service, in turn, is viewed as nonstigmatizing because the person or persons who provide it are valued and trusted by the community. As will be addressed in chapter 9, barbershops, for example, too, represent a vast untapped resource for reaching out to older adult men of color (Delgado, 2006). These establishments, however, present the field of health promotion with a different set of challenges when compared with their female counterparts in beauty parlors. Men, for example, spend less time in barbershops when compared with women in beauty parlors, making delivery of health education and screening more difficult to accomplish.

QUALITIES OF EFFECTIVE HEALTH PROMOTION PROGRAMS

Perkins, Simmett, and Wright (1999a,b) in their book on health promotion and evidence-based practice, highlight the rewards, challenges, and tensions of utilizing best practice evidence in the design, implementation, and evaluation of health promotion interventions. Raphael (2000) echoes many of the themes raised by Perkins, Simmett, and Wright (1999b), but also emphasizes the importance of ideology, values, and principles, shaping health promotion activities and efforts to measure their success and the need to be open to new ways of learning:

> In conclusion, it is important to recognize that the quality of evidence is influenced by a range of conceptual and technical factors. To date, it has generally been believed that only traditional or instrumental forms of knowledge are valid. Alternative forms of knowledge are as valid as—or even more valid—than traditional approaches for the kinds of issues health promoters deal with. It is important that various forms of evidence be collected, documented and shared with others in health promotion (p. 365).

Bunde-Birouste (2002, p. 6) summarized the current debates on health promotion effectiveness and concluded that they covered a wide range of topics: "Current debates about evidence encompass a broad range of questions: They range from debates on what sort of evidence is most relevant to different situations, capturing both qualitative and quantitative methods in health promotion programs and their implications, to the types of research methods used when compiling evidence." Bunde-Birouste's list is quite formidable in composition and serves notice to the field of health promotion not to be complacent and rest upon its laurels, significant as they may be.

Murphy (2005), in a comprehensive review of the international literature on health promotion, identified eleven recommendations for designing effective programs that resonate with much of what has been addressed in this book:

1. be specific in defining the health problem to be addressed and the key stakeholders at every relevant level
2. utilize behavioral theories as a guide
3. develop an in-depth understanding of the reasons for the health problem, with particular attention to barriers and vulnerabilities to achieving goals
4. involve stakeholders and community throughout all facets of an intervention
5. develop appropriate collaborations and pay close attention to practical aspects of planning
6. involve local role models in the programming
7. engage in capacity enhancement and be willing to involve and coordinate sector efforts
8. plan for a multifaceted intervention
9. work to increase the likelihood of sustainability by identifying and building upon community
10. evaluate using participatory and qualitative methods; this must be an integral part of programming
11. create participation and build a foundation to help ensure adaptation for future efforts

Each of these eleven recommendations brings with it a unique set of sociopolitical considerations with far-reaching implications for the field of health promotion, regardless of the characteristics of the population group it targets.

Kahan and Goodstadt (2001), for example, have raised a perspective on health promotion best practices that rarely gets raised. The authors argue that health promotion effectiveness can only be achieved through a reflective or interactional model and must build upon many of the concerns raised by Boutilier, Cleverly, and Labonte (2000):

Within health promotion, practice is not fixed by any rigorously defined discipline, and is said to be practiced by individuals in diverse organizations, training in a multiplicity of disciplines. Thus, what actually constitutes practice in health promotion will differ according to the practitioner's institutional location and discipline-related training, i.e., his or her "arena" of practice (p. 257).

Consequently, health promotion practice, like other forms of interdisciplinary practice such as youth development, is faced with a "moving target" of what constitutes health promotion ("Evidence in health promotion," 2003).

DEFINING HEALTH

There is a strong cultural dimension to any definition of health that must be taken into consideration in conceptualizing health promotion interventions (Benisovich & King, 2003; Garroutte, Sarkisian, Arguelles, Goldberg, & Buchwald, 2006). Gordon (2004) notes that race and ethnicity play a powerful role in shaping culture, as do other factors. However, the field must endeavor to avoid stereotyping as an expedient means of incorporating cultural factors into interventions. Simply noting the racial and ethnic background of older adults is insufficient to take into account how these factors influence their definition of health. This approach simply reinforces conventional stereotypes and does little to inform health care providers as to the actual meaning of health and the manifestations it takes on a daily basis in the life of older adults and their significant social networks.

As a result, health promotion interventions must take into account the sociocultural context upon which health is defined if these interventions are to be effective, particularly in the case of newcomers to the United States. This cultural dimension, however, goes far beyond conventional viewpoints that focus on culture as it relates to race and ethnicity. Guralnick (2003) rightly stresses the need for the field to develop greater awareness and skill in integrating cultural factors into interventions:

> Although opportunities to improve health promotion interventions for older adults abound, cultural differences can and do present major barriers to effective health care interventions. This is especially true when health practitioners overlook, misinterpret, stereotype, or otherwise mishandle their encounters with those who might be viewed as different from them in their assessment, intervention, and planning process. . . . (p. 2)

Garroutte and colleagues (2006) found in their study of older adult Native Americans that they often perceive their health status differently from that of their providers, raising the need for the field to reconcile these discordant perceptions. A. M. Miller and Iris (2002) found in their study of older adult definitions of health that four elements influence older adult perceptions of health: (1) functional independence, (2) self-care management of illness, (3) positive outlook on life, and (4) personal growth and social contribution. Each of these dimensions of health, in turn, influences health behaviors and shapes health promotion strategies for maintaining health. It is not unusual to find, as the reader will see in the following material, older adults, particularly those from the nondominant groups, who emphasize a holistic view of health.

Armer and Radina's (2002) study of Amish definitions of health and health promoting behaviors, for example, found that their religious and cultural beliefs influence how health is defined and addressed, highlighting significant differences between this group and the dominant American cultural views of health. The Amish use self-care practices such as liniments, vitamins, reflexology, midwives, therapeutic touch, and "Pow wowing," which is the use of sympathy curing utilizing words, charms, and physical manipulation. The authors uncovered six key themes, or dimensions, to defining health among the Amish: (1) the importance of achieving health, (2) an ability to work hard, (3) a sense of freedom to enjoy life, (4) family responsibility, (5) physical well-being, and (6) spiritual well-being.

Maddox (1999), in a study focused on older women and the social construction of health, identifies five themes related to the meaning of health for these women: (1) interactions with a greater being (spiritual); (2) acceptance of self; (3) possession of a sense of humor; (4) flexibility in life; and (5) being other-centered. Maddox (1999) concluded that it was essential that partnerships between providers and consumers were necessary to improve the quality of health care:

> Perhaps it is time to encourage older adults to become more of a partner in their care. . . . Health care professionals must continue to ask older adults about their view of health and encourage their partnership in health-related issues . . . by including older adults in the decision making process, this partnership should be strengthened (p. 32).

McVittie and Willock (2006), in turn, bring a different dimension to culture and health when they examine how health, ill health, and the concept of masculinity among older men influence a definition of what constitutes health. The authors, like their counterparts who studied women, concluded that social constructions of masculinity influence perceptions of health and help-seeking patterns. Clearly, gender brings an added dimension to any discussion of culture and older adults of color.

The National Research Council (Bulatao & Anderson, 2004), in a book titled *Understanding Racial and Ethnic Differences in Health in Late Life: A Research Agenda*, highlight four general ways how health promotion could result in different outcomes depending upon racial and ethnic cultural backgrounds of older adults:

1. health promotion influences help-seeking patterns
2. patient responses and perceptions of interventions may differ
3. the role of social environment/social network may enhance or detract from an intervention
4. alternative therapies such as folk medicine, which is heavily grounded within a cultural beliefs context, may produce different health outcomes

Finally, Falk, Sobal, Bisogni, Connors, and Devine (2001) approach health from an eating perspective and stressed the need for developing a definition of healthy eating by utilizing a multideterminant, context-dependent grounding that employs psychological, social, and cultural perspectives. A propensity to use simplified heuristics to deal with complex situations such as classification of foods into "healthy" and "unhealthy" categories is seriously deficient. Belief systems influence eating habits, like the broader construct of health, and must be understood in order to develop health promotion efforts and reduce professional role confusion. Falk and colleagues go on to emphasize that most health education campaigns are often based on professional definitions and not those of consumers, thereby undermining any efforts to achieve positive changes in healthy behavior.

Recognizing that there are major differences among older adults of color is an important initial step in making health promotion efforts group specific. However, Gelfand (2003) notes:

> Health promotion literature recognizes the importance of differences among the ethnic aged . . . but fails to provide substantial advice about techniques that are needed for effective health promotion with different ethnic groups. It is thus difficult to determine whether a therapeutic health program . . . which proves to be effective with African American elderly, would be equally effective, without revision, for elderly from other ethnic backgrounds (p. 147).

McMullen and Luborsky (2006) conclude that self-rated health appraisal among older adult African Americans is a complex process that is greatly influenced by the "sociohistorical content of individual assessments of well-being."

Use of self-rated health measures among Latino older adults as a means of better understanding definitions of health is also complex and must take into account acculturation level. Finch, Hummer, Reindi, and Vega (2002), for example, conclude based upon their study of the validity of self-rated health among Latinos that the use of self-rated health to assess physical health must control for levels of acculturation. Somatization of emotional/mental health, for example, is influenced by acculturation level. Health promotion efforts targeting Latino older adults, as a consequence, cannot ignore the interaction of acculturation and self-rated health.

The complexity of a cultural construct is intertwined with the complexity of health, particularly when it is defined to take into account the interplay of social, cultural, and economic systems. McCarthy, Ruiz, Gale, Karam, and Moore (2004) explore the cultural meaning of health among older Latina and white non-Latinas. Their qualitative study's findings highlight the vast differences in how these two groups define and perceive "functional" health. The authors stress the deleterious consequences of ethnocentrism in expectations of health and help seeking and, indirectly, health promotion practice.

The subject of acculturation and Latino older adults has generally been overlooked in the field, although acculturation measures have much to offer health promotion initiatives (Chiriboga, 2004). Yamada, Valle, Barrio, and Jeste (2006), in a rare article specifically focused on acculturation measures and Latino older adults, conclude that this population group has generally been overlooked in the research literature and is worthy of having acculturation measures specifically developed for them. The authors identified four specific contexts in which aging and acculturation intersect, with implications for research and service delivery to Latino older adults: (1) impact of aging on acculturation, (2) degree of pressure to assimilate during late life, (3) impact of the role of older Latinos on acculturation, and (4) opportunities for assimilation or biculturation. Gonzalez, Haan, and Hinton (2001), for example, found a higher level of depression among the least acculturated older Mexican Americans (aged sixty to one hundred), and this represents one of the many ways that acculturation can be systematically applied to multiple arenas with implications for health promotion.

It is not unusual to associate a list of health problems, or ailments, when discussing health promotion and Latino older adults. As already noted in chapter 4, they certainly face a range of challenges in narrowing the gap in health disparities. Nevertheless, in the case of Latino older adults, there are significant forces operating that result in positive health outcomes, resulting in health promotion initiatives identifying these forces and incorporating them in interventions. There is a longevity difference between Latino older adults who are newcomers to the United States and those born and raised in the United States or who have resided in the country for a long period of time. This difference persists even when the newcomer is of lower socioeconomic status and received less formal health care over their lifetime (Kolata, 2007). Not surprisingly, there has been an emerging debate about what is referred to as the "Hispanic health paradox." This debate, however, has implications for health promotion that go far beyond academic interests and touch upon a variety of important factors related to the Latino older adult community, health, and health promotion.

Haywood, Warner, and Crimmins' (2007, p. 93) study of native-born Mexican Americans found that connectivity does not translate into less likelihood of being disabled when compared with white non-Latinos: "On the whole, we do not find much evidence to support the idea of an Hispanic paradox with respect to disability among native-born Mexican-Americans. While Mexican-Americans and whites share life chances, they have different disability experiences over their lifetimes." Markides and colleagues (2007), however, found no immigrant advantage over native-born Mexican Americans in lower rates of either premature or incidence of disability among Latinos in the United States. Pulloni (2007) argues that the Hispanic health paradox is a "scientific" problem that is unsolvable at this point in time because of structural and methodological shortcomings.

R. J. Martinez's (1999) ethnographic research on the health of older Latinos in Southern Colorado found three important cultural domains related to definitions of health: (1) health is creating balance in life by living one's beliefs, (2) health is maintained by successfully fulfilling one's obligations to others, and (3) health is faith that one will be cared for by God, family, and community. Martinez (1999, p. 1) goes on to note: "Participants held holistic views of self and spiritual aspects of life played a major role in their health. Caring for self was lived through caring for others for whom one has responsibility." The degree of interconnectedness with others clearly was central to how this group of older Latinos viewed health.

The construct of spirituality is often found alongside that of culture for very good reasons. These two constructs are closely intertwined and wield great influence on one another. Wycherley (2001) and Nash (2001) contribute a different perspective than the one usually associated with the topic of religion and health. The spiritual self, or holistic self, brings a dimension to older adult health promotion that is not necessarily tied to a "greater being" but does connect them to the "greater good." A holistic perspective brings the field of older adult health promotion an opportunity to expand conventional views, and it allows the introduction of innovative strategies that capitalize on these constructs. How spirituality or a holistic perspective is viewed may well differ among and within older adult racial and ethnic groups, necessitating that every effort be made to identify this definition before development of a health promotion effort.

King, Burgess, Akinyela, Courts-Spriggs, and Parker (2005) examine the role of spirituality in shaping health beliefs among African-American older adults and found that it has significant influences in defining health. Polzer and Miles (2007) found spirituality to be an important factor in how African Americans self-manage their diabetes. Almqvist, Hellnas, Stefansson, and Granlund (2006), in turn, examine perceptions and definitions of health from a young child's (four to five years old) perspective and address the role of play in child engagement in health promotion efforts targeting young children. Innovative efforts such as this are also needed at the opposite end of the age continuum. Incentives to participate in health promotion efforts must be created that are culture bound and sensitive to the beliefs and attitudes of older adults from non–Western European backgrounds.

Damron-Rodríguez, Frank, Enríquez-Haass, and Reuben (2005) examine similarities and differences of definitions of health among different older adult ethnic groups (African Americans, Chinese, Eastern Europeans, and Latinos) and concluded that cultural aspects wield a tremendous amount of influence in shaping older adult perceptions of their health. They note (2005):

> Biopsychosocial and spiritual dimensions of health are not routinely part of how most health professions frame health promotion for older adults. Additionally, older adults' perceptions of health appear to be based on a strengths model, while assessment by health professionals is founded in a problem-based model (p. 15).

Consequently, the importance of health promotion strategies' taking into account how a group defines health, and the multifaceted set of factors that enter into this definition, take on prominence and raise the importance of culture in dictating definition and interventions.

Henderson and Ainsworth (2003), for example, in their qualitative study of older African American and American Indian women and their perceptions of physical activity, found that most perceived themselves to be very active physically and that these perceptions were greatly influenced by personal and cultural values. Tudor-Locke and colleagues (2003), in turn, stress the importance of tapping the voices of African American and Native American women in defining and interpreting what is meant by physical activity. For example, the concept of "leisure" may be interpreted as "laziness."

Armer and Radina's (2002) findings pertaining to the Amish, like the others presented in this section, highlight the multifaceted dimension of health among nondominant groups in this society. Healthy well-being goes far beyond a physical state or the absence of illness and disease. The sociocultural dimensions of health require the field of health promotion to develop interventions that systematically tap a group's definition of health. This obviously complicates the process and makes it both labor and time intensive. It also highlights the advantages of older adults them-selves playing a critical role in both the conceptualization of the goals of health promotion and also the most appropriate methods for delivering content. Older adult-led health promotion, as a result, has the philosophi-cal underpinnings for taking into account group-specific conceptions of health and health promoting behaviors.

Culturally grounding health definitions and actions represent a critical step in making health care, including health promotion, contextualized to take into account the definitions and perceptions of health held by histori-cally undervalued groups in this society. Definitions and interpretations of perceptions, as a result, are socially and culturally constructed and must be taken into account in the development of any health promotion initiative targeting older adults, particularly those of color (Henderson & Ainsworth, 2000). The voices of those being targeted need to influence how health, as in this case involving physical activity, gets defined. Older adult-led health promotion is fundamentally based upon empowering older adults, and this can only be successfully accomplished when their voices (beliefs, perceptions, desires) are systematically taken into account in the construction of this social intervention.

COMPLEMENTARY AND ALTERNATIVE MEDICINE

Any discussion of older adult health promotion would not be com-plete without a discussion of complementary and alternative medicine. Becker, Gates and Newsom (2004), although referring to self-care, make an important observation and provide an important rationale for why complementary and alternative medicine exists, and why they wield such tremendous influence within circles of older adults of color:

> Underlying culturally based self-care practices are important not only in gen-eral; they give rise to the development of illness-specific self-care schemes for chronic illnesses. However, regardless of the sophistication of biomedically influenced self-care schemes that people may evolve, cultural approaches to self-care are ongoing and an intrinsic part of daily life. Those approaches not only form the precursor to the incorporation of biomedically derived self-care approaches, they offer a complementary philosophy that both enhances the incorporation of these approaches and interacts with them, as others have also found (p. 2072).

Cherniack, Senzel, and Pan (2001) found complementary and alterna-tive medicine to be highly prevalent among a sample of New York City older adults, particularly among females and those with higher formal levels of education. One recent study, however, found that middle-aged adults are more likely to utilize complementary and alternative medicine than their older adult counterparts (Middle-aged adults, 2007). Consequently, the use of complementary and alternative medicine should not be considered the exclusive purview of low-income older adults with limited access to quality health care. Use of self-prayer, however, is a method used almost exclusively by older adults.

Montalto, Bhargava, and Hong (2006) recommend that the field of health promotion undertake more qualitative studies to develop further insights into the use of complementary and alternative medicine use by older adults. R. J. Cohen, Kirsten, and Pan (2002) recommend that information on complementary and alternative medicine be systematically gathered by physicians in order to help ensure quality service delivery and to enhance our understanding about drug-herb/drug-supplement interactions. Arcury and colleagues (2007), for example, found that herbs played a central role in health self-management among older adults, with use being greatly influenced by cultural and personal resources. Ford's (2000) study of older African-American women and their natural health-helping resources, found that religious institutions, extended family and friends, and complementary and alternative medicines were instrumental parts of this network. Bell and colleagues (2006), in turn, found complementary and alternative medicine use high among older adults with hypertension.

There certainly are a variety of ways that health promotion programs can take into account and possibly integrate indigenous healing into programming and activities. R. J. Martinez (1999), for example, makes an important recommendation for the role of health providers/promoters regarding how best to approach and assess the role of remedies among older adults, particularly in the case of those who do not share a Western view of the world, such as Latinos:

> Many of these care providers were Hispanics, from the region, and able to discuss *remedios* openly with patients they served. While *remedios* allowed people to care for themselves and each other in a convenient, affordable, and culturally acceptable way, it is important to recognize the possibility of adverse drug interactions when patients use both remedies and prescription medications. There is a potential danger that some patients, fearing that the doctor will ask them to stop, or that their traditional treatments will be devalued, may not inform their doctor about use of remedies. As more knowledge is gained about the herbs that are used in folk medicine, pharmacists should be able to advise doctors in this area (p. 47).

Hill (2003), based upon a study of health promotion and complementary and alternative medicine providers, concludes that collaboration between these two perspectives on health care was not only possible but also highly advisable, if they both embrace education and empowerment models. Health promoters who are committed to social action, however, offer the greatest promise for achieving this form of collaboration. Complementary and alternative medicine is closely associated with cultural conceptions and definitions of health and represents a critical way in which older adults practice self-care. It would be foolish to ignore this perspective in any serious effort at development of culturally competent forms of health promotion.

THEORIES OF HEALTH BEHAVIOR

Health behavior theory, simply stated, represents an integrated set of propositions and beliefs that seek to explain a phenomenon—in the case of this book, older adult health. The role and importance of theory guiding how health promotion gets conceptualized and implemented is well understood in the field. Nutbeam and Harris (1999), however, make the observation that theories used to build health promotion initiatives are often more implicit than explicit in how they shape an intervention.

S. C. Jones and Donovan (2004), in their review of health promotion theories used in Australia, found that a wide mixture of theories could be found in the field, with precede-proceed and the transtheoretical (stages of change) models being used by almost one-third of all sampled practitioners. Cottrell and colleagues (2002, p. 101) rightly surmise that "good" health promotion programs are not the result of luck: "Good health promotion programs are not created by chance. They are the result of much hard work and are organized around a well-thought-out and well conceived model." McKenzie and Smeltzer (2001), in turn, bring a different dimension to the discussion of health behavior theories by stressing the importance of planning:

> The effectiveness of health promotion programs can vary greatly. However, the success of a program can usually be linked to the planning [theory informed] that takes place before implementation of the program. Programs that have undergone a thorough planning process are usually the most successful. As the old saying goes, "If you fail to plan, your plan will fail" (p. 4–5)

Health promotion theories of behavior not only guide practitioners and academics in implementing and evaluating programs, but they also help move the field forward by facilitating communication about activities and serve as the basis for introduction of innovative thinking on how health promotion should evolve in the future. Theories of health behavior are often considered the foundation for any health promotion initiative, and as a result, are considered pivotal in conceptualizing health promotion regardless of the group being addressed. In the case of older adults, however, these theories take into account development/life span dimensions and seek to ground experiences about health within a social context.

Bandura (2004), for example, advances a multifaceted causal structure that highlights how self-efficacy beliefs and actions affect personal health habits. Purdie and McCrindle (2002) explore self-regulation (purposeful, strategic, and persistence in undertaking action), self-efficacy, and human behavior change in older adults, and conclude that there is a strong relationship between self-efficacy (confidence) and self-regulation (action) in addressing health and health behaviors among older adults. This relationship, in turn, must be systematically integrated into health promotion efforts that specifically target this population group. Health promotion programs that rely heavily upon messages and tactics that stress vulnerability and severity tend to also negate self-efficacy and thereby are destined to be of limited effectiveness in reaching older adults (Murphy & Bennett, 2002). As noted in the following chapter, self-efficacy and self-care are also strongly associated and bring an important cultural dimension to older adult health promotion that offers the potential for innovative ways of increasing consumer participation in this form of health promotion.

There are certainly no absences of theories of behavior informing health promotion interventions (Perkins et al., 1999a). Bandura (2004) argues, like many other scholars, that human health is a social matter and not just an individual matter, thereby opening up numerous interpretations and approaches toward addressing ill health. Nutbeam and Harris's (1999) conclusions concerning theories of health promotion represent my own views, as well as those of countless others in the field:

> There is no single theory or model that can adequately guide the development of a comprehensive health promotion program intended to influence the multiple determinants of health in populations. Practitioners need to use local knowledge and experience, and available research information to make judgments about community needs and the determinants of health that are most amenable to change at any particular time (p. 75–76).

It is clear that the field does not subscribe to any one theory concerning health and health promotion. However, health promotion theories generally fall into three categories depending upon the emphasis they place on individuals, organizations, and communities (Health Promotion Agency, 2007). This book, as the reader no doubt surmises, bridges all three arenas in how older adult-led health promotion conceptualizes health promotion. This section will only provide the reader with a brief summary of the most relevant theories that guide older adult-led health promotion.

(1) Theories that focus their attention on explaining health behaviors by focusing on individuals have wielded considerable influence in guiding

most health promotion theories, and this book on older adult-led health promotion is certainly no exception. Theories such as health beliefs theory of reasoned action, transtheoretical (stages of change), and social learning theory probably represent the most significant examples. However, social learning theory is arguably the most prevalent theory, and that is why it is highlighted in this section.

Social Learning Theory: The importance of social learning theory is well established. However, it takes on great significance when applied to urban communities because of the close proximity of living arrangements and the concentration of people who live within a prescribed geographical boundary. Social learning theory places great importance on the observation and modeling of behaviors and attitudes (Galea & Vlahov, 2005). Thus, health promotion initiatives and programs predicated on contagiousness of ideas and social examples generally have social learning theory as a strong foundation. Belyea, Pierce, and Lamwi-Keefe (2003) note that social learning theory lends itself to engaging participants in more effectively overcoming obstacles and better appreciating their success in doing so, by addressing three critical dimensions:

> (1) personal factors, such as attitudes and value; (2) environmental influences, such as social relationships and physical environment; and (3) factors associated with the behavior itself, such as perceived capability to perform the behavior and outcomes expected for performing the behavior (p. 737).

Social learning theory, not surprisingly, has played a highly prominent role within health promotion, particularly when viewed from a peer-to-peer intervention perspective (D. L. Baker, 2001). However, this theory has largely been devoted to setting a foundation for peer-driven health promotion involving youth. Its applicability, nevertheless, is not restricted to youth and can also be applied to older adults and other population groups. For example, the use of older adults as peer providers of health promotion and other services is not new to the field of gerontology, as already noted in chapter 1. The concept of peer educator/counselor has a long history within the health promotion field. However, peer education has generally been limited to select age groups with particular emphasis on youth. Nevertheless, the use of peer education is not inherently restricted for use with older adults.

The 1970s and 1980s, for example, evidenced a substantial body of scholarly literature on older adults as "peer counselors." This literature highlighted older adult contributions in the areas of nutrition, loneliness, bereavement, nursing home care, and recovery from illness, for example (Chapman & Pancoast, 1985; E. M. Gallagher, 1985; Ho et al., 1987; Lynde, 1992; Milligan, Maryland, Ziegler, & Ward, 1987; Sutherland, Cowar, & Heck, 1988; Weinrich, Weinrich, Stromborg, Boyd, & Weiss, 1993). An eleven-page annotated bibliography on this early period literature attests to the popularity of the concept (Peer Resources, n.d.). Most of this literature, unfortunately, did not address older adults of color, with notable exceptions. More recently, the Texas Cooperative Extension (2006) reports on an older adult peer education program. Gordon (2004) recommends hiring older adults as consultants to programs as a means of both increasing the likelihood of success for these programs and empowering older adults in the process.

In summary, Nutbeam and Harris (2003) are not surprised by the popularity of social learning theory and health promotion:

> Not surprisingly, a review of health promotion literature in the past decade reveals a large number of health promotion interventions that combine educational programs with modification of the social and physical environments based on social cognition theory. This continuous "field testing" adds further confidence to the usefulness of this theory to guide practice (p. 22).

Social learning theory lends itself quite well to being integrated into comprehensive health promotion programs, such as the one being advocated for in this book.

(2) Theories that focus on communities and community actions have also increasingly gained popularity as the field of health promotion has expanded its reach into macro-arenas; community mobilization (social planning, social action, community development) and diffusion of innovation best typify the approaches toward health promotion taken by this genre. These theories stand out in importance regarding older adult-led health promotion, explaining why they are the focus in this book.

Erben, Franzkowiak, and Wenzel (2000) argue that the Ottawa Charter effectively aimed at various levels of collective action intended to improve health at both the individual and collective levels. Laverack (2004, p. 33) argues that empowerment is "at the heart of the 'new' health promotion, and power is at the core of empowerment." Empowerment is a critical concept central to the vision of health promotion embodied by the Ottawa Charter. J. L. Collins, Giles, and Holmes-Chavez (2007, p. A42), reporting on the recommendations of the National Expert Panel on Community Health Promotion (Centers for Disease Control and Prevention's National Center for Chronic Disease Prevention and Health Promotion), offer a number of recommendations, with one being "to increase the effects of public health programs by seeking expanded skills and expertise in the theory and practice of social change and working to integrate that expertise into public health practice."

The role and influence of social environment on health, particularly in cases where social structure systematically undermines health through exposure to toxic substances, lack of access to quality care, and introduction of stress, must be instrumental in any concerted effort to address health in economically marginalized urban communities. Our ability to balance individual needs without losing sight of the broader social forces and their impact on health and help seeking will no doubt remain a perennial challenge for the field of health promotion. These change-oriented theories seek to combine individual and community-focused empowerment. Empowerment with the purposes of achieving public policy changes to enhance health invariably involve three critical components (Nathonson, 1999):

1. the emergence of a scientifically and socially recognized threat to public health,
2. the ability to identify and mobilize a constituency that involves multiple organizational and community entities
3. the mergence of political opportunities with target-group vulnerabilities

Theories on change in communities bring to health promotion three perspectives that are complementary with each other but also support social learning theory (Nutbeam & Harris, 2003, p. 25): "1. Introducing new ideas into communities (diffusion of innovation); 2. Identifying key approaches by organizations and workers to bring about change in local communities (community organization); and 3. Making communities more central in decisions about their futures (community building)." The relationship between health promotion, empowerment, and community development has its share of advocates in the field, including myself (Chappell, Funk, Carson, MacKenzie, & Stanwick, 2006). Goodstadt (2007), for example, advocates for the merging of community development and health promotion constructs as a means of improving the health of communities and increasing their capacities to do so in the future as well.

Delgado and Zhou (2008), in their book titled *Youth-Led Health Promotion in Urban Communities: A Community Capacity-Enhancement Perspective*, stress the use of theories on community change to argue for the importance of health promotion being viewed from a lens that goes far beyond the individual to include families, communities, and the organizations within communities. Mobilizing communities not only define their assets and health problems, and thereby shape the nature of interventions, but also play decision making roles in how interventions are to be conceptualized and evaluated and applied to youth, adults, and older adults, as in the case of this book. Theories on community change actively seek to increase participation and integrate empowerment goals. The process of arriving at a health promotion strategy that is culturally competent is as important, and some would argue more important, than the actual delivery of health promotion.

Margen and Lashof's (2000, p. 699) charge to the field of public health, and health promotion as a significant part of this field, resonates well with the central thrust and goals of this book and makes a fitting theoretical foundation for older adult-led health promotion: "As public health professionals, we must not isolate ourselves from society, rather, we must become activists for social change that will result in equity for all while still acknowledging the uniqueness of each individual. This must be our goal for the millennium. How far we can progress depends on how well we learn to work together."

The reader has every right to ask what makes the model of older adult-led health promotion so different, if at all, from that which was practiced over twenty years ago when peer-led models pertaining to older adults were popular across the United States. As already noted in chapter 1, the answer lies in the emergence and configuration of a set of values, principles, strategies, and activities that place older adults front and center in this intervention, and the significance of social context in shaping this form of health promotion. Central to older adult-led health promotion is an embrace of social and economic justice values and perspectives, as the reader will see in the next chapter. This element, unfortunately, was not a critical element in most forms of peer counseling involving older adults in the 1970s and 1980s. Older adult-led health promotion, as noted in the following chapter and previous sections of this book, targets individuals, organizations, communities, and social policies. As a result, such an approach toward health promotion must draw upon multiple theories to guide actions.

This section has hopefully provided the reader with an understanding of several different theoretical approaches that older adult-led health promotion relies upon to shape assessment, intervention, and evaluation of efforts. These and other less well-known theories have started to gain increasing applicability when applied to older adults and the unique circumstances and challenges that they face.

HEALTH LITERACY

Health promotion, as the reader has no doubt surmised by now, comprises a multitude of dimensions, perspectives, and subjects. However, the role of health literacy invariably plays an influential role in any way health promotion gets defined because of the central role that language plays in this subject matter (Aspinalla, 2007; Lloyd, Ammary, Epstein, Johnson, & Rhee, 2006). In fact, it is rare for any serious discussion of older adult health promotion to take place without the subject of health literacy emerging as an important dimension of any health promotion initiative.

There certainly is no shortage of how health literacy has been defined in the field. However, older adult health literacy can be simply defined as the abilities of older adults to "obtain, interpret and understand basic health information and services, and the competency and motivation to apply generalized information to personal situations" (Dorsett, 2004, p. 1). Literacy generally gets classified as prose, document, or quantitative. Health literacy, in turn, is viewed from three domains or dimensions: (1) clinical, (2) prevention, and (3) navigation of the health care system (Kutner, Greenberg, Jin, & Paulsen 2006). The relationship between health promotion, health literacy, and cultural competency is quite evident in any serious effort to effectively disseminate intended messages (Dorsett, 2004). This subject matter increases in significance when discussing older adults of color who do not have English as their primary language (Aspinalla, 2007).

A 2003 study of health literacy of America's adult population found that adults age sixty-five years and older had lower average health literacy than younger adult age groups (Kutner et al., 2006). Wallace (2004), in turn, challenges the field to develop health promotion materials that are both linguistically and culturally appropriate for older adults with low formal education and English not their primary language. Sudore and colleagues (2006) concluded that limited literacy is common, but its prevalence increases with age and is independently associated with a 200 percent increase in mortality among older adults.

Low health literacy among older adults, for example, predicts higher mortality rates (D. W. Baker, Gazmararian, Sudano, & Patterson, 2000), higher mortality cardiovascular deaths (D. W. Baker et al., 2000, 2007), higher hospitalization rates (D. W. Baker et al., 2007), severe health consequences due to poor adherence and inappropriate use of medications (Roth & Ivey, 2005), and poor physical functioning and mental health (S. Y. D. Lee, Gazmararian, Arozullah, & Brown, 2006; Wolf, Gazmararian, & Baker, 2005). Consequently, health literacy is not restricted to any one facet of health promotion or setting but has particular applicability to older adults, particularly those with limited English proficiency.

McCray (2005), in an extensive review of the literature on health literacy, advocates for greater attention being paid to this subject in an effort to develop greater knowledge of the complex interactions between "general literacy, health-literacy, information technologies, and the existing health care infrastructure." Health literacy, as a result, must be highly contextualized to the population group being targeted by health promotion in order to utilize cultural symbols and language to better reach older adults with overall low literacy rates.

The older adult health promotion effort described by Valle, Yamada, and Matiella (2006) captures the spirit and need for innovative approaches to increase health literacy from a culturally competent viewpoint. The authors utilized *fotonovelas* (soap operas) to reach Latino older adults and increase their knowledge of Alzheimer's disease and related disorders. A soap opera format taps into the popularity of *novelas* as an entertainment medium among Latinos.

SOCIAL JUSTICE AND ENVIRONMENTAL HEALTH

The emergence of environmental social justice has managed to capture the attention and imagination of various groups, most notably youth (Delgado & Zhou, 2008; Quiroz-Martinez et al., 2005). Schulz and Northridge (2004) conclude, based on their study of social determinants of health and environmental health promotion, that interventions must anticipate political and economic challenges and unintentional consequences. The authors also issue a call for broadening and engaging those "outside of the health sector" to enter into collaborations to improve the health of communities exposed to toxic environmental pollutants. Bringing attention to the social determinants of health regarding environmental factors has expanded the field of health promotion to encompass the broader community and shifted focus away from individual risk factors (Brown, 2007; Howze, Baldwin, & Kegler, 2004; Kreuter, Rosa, Howze, & Baldwin, 2004; Schulz & Northridge, 2004). Nevertheless, environmental justice is not restricted to youth and can find relevance across the life cycle, including among older adults.

Older adult-led health promotion transpires with a keen understanding of how environment shapes health. Environmental hazards affect older adults of color in a variety of ways depending upon geographical location. Markey (2003) provides three such examples that illustrate how ethnicity/racial and geographical context relates to environmental health:

Older African American residents of West Oakland, Calif., may not know what vinyl chloride is, but many were relieved when the Red Star Yeast/Lasaffre plant in their neighborhood closed last April. American Indian elders in California's Pitt River Region are worried about high levels of inorganic mercury poisoning dating back to the California Gold Rush when mercury was used for mining, as well as deposits from batteries, thermometers and other devices currently dumped in their area. Low-income Latino elders in the Central San Joaquin Valley community of Peterson are not only concerned about pesticides, but they also report that their grandchildren must wear high boots on rainy days because the sewage system is so old it leaks raw effluent into the streets (p. 1).

The above three case examples come out of a qualitative study specifically focused on older adults of color in California and environmental health. The study sought information on three critical items (Markey, 2003, p. 4): "1. Prioritize and study environmental health threats to older people. 2. Examine the effect that a rapidly growing aging population might have on our environment. 3. Encourage older adults to volunteer in their own communities to help reduce hazards and protect the environment." The uniqueness of this study and the findings reported make the subject of environmental health and health promotion highly relevant, with considerable potential to be an active form of older adult-led health promotion (Markey, 2003):

1. Participants want leadership training for community advocates.
2. Participants have a lack of trust in corporations and government officials.
3. Participants want an easy and accessible venue for lodging complaints against polluters, available in multiple languages.
4. Participants want more information about the environmental effects on health.
5. Participants believe the government should improve and enforce environmental regulations that are in the interest of residents.
6. Participants believe the polluting companies should be responsible for any medical expenses incurred as a result of environmental hazards.
7. Participants want improved warning times and devices for companies who discover there has been an environmental leak, explosion, etc.
8. Many participants work under illegal and unsafe conditions. They are not provided with the safety gear required to work in hazardous work environments.
9. Participants want young people to become involved. They say that younger people are usually less aware of problems than the older adults so there is an opportunity for older adults to teach young people.
10. The majority of community elders seemed willing to be involved in volunteering provided there was strong leadership to motivate them.
11. Some participants had other important issues to deal with, such as childrearing, other financial and health problems, volunteer commitments, etc., and did not believe that putting their energies towards fighting environmental injustice was a priority (p. 16).

The findings from the California study were reported to the Environmental Protection Agency. However, the implications go far beyond one governmental agency and highlight the potential for older adult participation and leadership in environmental health change efforts. Challenges were also uncovered. Competing demands, the need for leadership, and their own pressing health, economic, and social needs, for example, are not unique to this particular group of older adults. Not every older adult will see environmental health as a priority, and that is no different than any other age group. Nevertheless, there are some older adults who see it as a priority, and this group is ideal for engagement in older adult-led health promotion. The high percentage of older adults of color who have worked in industries where they have been exposed to toxic conditions and safety threats will see great value and meaning in environmental justice and health.

COMMUNITY HEALTH EDUCATION

Strategies can be defined as methods that have proven to be effective at achieving intervention goals across multiple interventions and replications (Brounstein, Gardner, & Backer, 2006). When examining strategies often found in delivering health promotion to urban-based older adults, the role and prominence of community health education stands out. The history of health education is one that predates health promotion, and it is one that reflects an embrace of a wide set of values and principles that make community health education an integral part of most health promotion definitions and strategies.

Health education that is community centered (namely, delivered within a community-based setting) is often an integral part of any older adult health promotion initiative. There is considerable flexibility in how health education gets conceptualized and implemented. It can take the shape of a one-time event, or it can be a series of educational events covering one or multiple topics. Further, the event can cover a relatively short time period or an extensive period with multiple breaks. This flexibility in how to conceptualize community health education makes it quite appealing to include this activity as part of a broader health promotion strategy.

States and colleagues (2006) report on the success of a series of community health education workshops targeting older adults of color in Brooklyn, New York. These workshops were titled "Understanding Dementia," "Living with Memory Changes," "Understanding Depression," and "Strategies for Change" and were designed to stand alone, be offered in multiple languages, and be based upon the cultural values of older adults in the community. Community health education workshops can be quite successful in achieving health promotion goals when conducted in a culturally competent manner. This, in turn, does require these workshop sessions to be conducted in community-based settings that are easily accessible geographically, operationally, psychologically, and culturally.

The social context of health and health promotion serves to increase the importance of health and health promotion being grounded within a cultural context that takes into account older adult perceptions. These expectations systematically incorporate values and belief systems to increase the likelihood that an intervention is welcomed. Having said this, however, means that academics and practitioners understand and embrace a socioecological perspective on health promotion targeting older adults, and more so in cases where this form of intervention is focused on marginalized older adults of color.

Healthy aging must be conceptualized as the rule rather than the exception (Himes, 2002). The potential of health promotion to prevent certain illnesses or minimize complications when these illnesses occur provides the field with a wide range of possibilities for constructing interventions across a spectrum of social arenas. Older adult-led health promotion, in turn, brings with it the potential to empower older adults and enhance community capacity in the process. A multifaceted vision of health promotion, as a result, facilitates the creation of partnerships between consumers, professionals, and indigenous providers.

6

*

Older Adult-Led
Health Promotion

"It is often said that we live in an aging world. This fact represents one
of the major success stories of the 20th century, but simultaneously
presents the 21st century with one of its major challenges."

(Beck, 2000, p. 424)

There is a general understanding that an increase in life longevity is
often a criterion used to determine the health and progress of a society
(Breslaw, 2000; Nakasato & Carnes, 2006). However, with an increased life
expectancy comes a host of challenges for all fields, particularly the health
field because of its potential role in helping to prevent and treat illnesses
and diseases that can shorten a life span and increase well-being (Beck,
2000; CDC, 2005; Duxbury, 2000; Resnick, 2001a). This criterion also brings
increased expectations for social interventions such as health promotion to
help older adults live a healthier and better life (Beattie, Whitelaw, Mettler,
& Turner, 2003). Values pertaining to the importance of increased health
well-being may, in part, be fueled by concerns about escalating costs of
medical care for this age group. However, bringing economic concerns to
the forefront rather than concerns about quality of life for older adults may
be a serious strategic mistake on the part of the field.

Richardson (2006) makes the observation that health promotion cannot
simply be applied across the life span without making necessary changes
to reflect the unique needs of different age groups and their social circumstances:

Promoting the health of older adults is not simply a matter of taking existing
guidelines and extrapolating them. . . . Older adults [present unique needs].

121

. . . Because of these factors, health promotion and disease prevention activities are forgotten or overlooked. On the other hand, overzealous healthcare professionals sometimes inappropriately apply recommendations developed for young or middle-aged adults to frail older adults with limited life expectancy (p. 1).

Richardson's (2006) call for age-group specific programming will not come as a surprise to the health promotion field, or any other field of practice, for that matter. Nevertheless, such a call may be considered labor intensive and, as a result, costly by policy makers because of the need to "individualize" initiatives to take into account age and, one might add, local social context as well.

Ruffing-Rahal (1991), in an article dating back to the early 1990s, specifically puts forth a model of health promotion for older adults that is multifaceted and multisetting focused, and can be considered ahead of its time because of how it stresses local context in setting a health promotion agenda: enhancement of self-care skills, emotional and spiritual integration, and social integration. The elements advanced in this model can easily be considered quite innovative by today's standards, and highlight the importance of taking a socioecological view of older adult health. Clearly, the importance of taking a holistic perspective (social, economic, political, and spiritual) enhances what is meant by a healthy state of being for older adults, and is very much in tone with the most progressive models on older adult health promotion being advocated in present day. The case study of Older Women's Network presented in chapter 10 typifies how a holistic perspective becomes operational.

As already noted in chapters 1 and 5, the health promotion field has expanded dramatically over the past decade to encompass a variety of perspectives, strategies, settings, and population groups. The very nature of how fast this field of practice has expanded attests to its potential and ability to dramatically alter health conditions in communities nationally and internationally (Delgado & Zhou, 2008; Saskatchewan Health, 2003). However, as to be expected with any rapid expansion of any social intervention, questions pertaining to nature, applicability, effectiveness, and boundaries are bound to emerge.

When research findings are available and can be translated into practice, it does not occur at the pace that both academics and practitioners want it to (Glasgow, Lichtenstein, & Marcus, 2003). Questions also arise as to who are, and who are not, benefiting from these interventions. Further, the question of who is "best" qualified to undertake health promotion with this population group has started to surface in both academic and practice arenas. This questioning has led rise to the possibility of older adults playing critical roles in shaping and carrying out health promotion initiatives.

PRINCIPLES

I have always found that subscribing to a set of principles for practice facilitates the integration of theory into the complex world of practice and makes engaging different parties and constituencies easier to accomplish. Principles do not originate out of thin air and can be considered representations of key values and theory, thereby acting as a bridge between the academic and practice worlds. The principles that follow are not by all means the only principles out in the world of health promotion and older adults. Minkler and Checkoway (1988), twenty years ago, articulated a set of ten principles that stressed empowerment and strengths, and not just needs, that should be the foundation of older adult health promotion. Endres and Holmes (2006–07), too, outlined a set of ten principles related to older adults. Their principles focused on older adult civic engagement, and like those of Minkler and Checkoway (1988), have found their way into this section and throughout this book in various forms and depth.

The following principles represent one individual's view; the reader, as to be expected, may agree with some or many of these principles and, of course, have other principles that they bring to this field. Having clarity about "what is important" facilitates collaboration across disciplines and with consumers. Consumers, too, will bring a set of principles to practice, although the wording of these principles will not be similar to that of academics. This does not mean that there cannot be overlaps as well as differences. A total of ten principles are presented. These principles are not presented in any order of priority, however, and it is left up to the reader to decide their priority based upon the local circumstances within which they are practicing.

1. Health promotion efforts must be grounded within the social context and operative reality of older adults. "One size" does not fit all, and local circumstances must dictate interventions and necessary modifications to national and international models of older adult-led health promotion. Flexibility in the conceptualizing of older adult health promotion must be encouraged in order for efforts to be tailored in a manner that is culturally affirming, thereby increasing the likelihood of acceptance by older adults and their communities.
2. Social and economic justice, and empowerment, must serve as the guiding forces in the design and implementation of older adult-led

health promotion. An ecological perspective on health and health inequities cannot be divorced from issues related to oppression of marginalized older adults. Empowerment, though an elusive and not universally defined construct, must still take a prominent place with older adult-led health promotion. Its definition and operations must be dictated by older adults and supported by organizations and staff.

3. Older adult-led health promotion must be multifaceted and address health at an individual, family, community, and societal level. This does not mean that efforts at addressing health promotion cannot start with the individual older adult. However, this represents a starting point rather than a destination. Ultimately, other levels must be addressed if the forces resulting in the health condition(s) being addressed are grounded upon discrimination based upon the beliefs and demographic characteristics of the older adults being targeted, necessitating an emphasis on social and economic justice values and principles guiding health promotion interventions.

4. Older adults and their respective communities must have their capacities enhanced throughout all facets of older adult-led health promotion since it is insufficient to have health promotion just focus on health. Community capacity enhancement represents a key element of healthy well-being, and as a result, must be a goal of any health promotion program. The broader community that older adults are a part of can, and should, be expected to benefit from health promotion led by older adults.

5. Older adult-led health promotion must actively seek to provide necessary educational, financial, and social support to facilitate participation of older adults regardless of their beliefs and social, economic, and physical circumstances. Inclusivity rather than exclusivity must be a central goal. Health, according to Given and Given (2001), needs to be conceptualized to include independence and function, and not just disease-free/illness-free status. This more encompassing perspective challenges the field of health promotion to develop strategies that systematically address a multitude of factors and levels that influence health and health-seeking behaviors.

6. Organizations sponsoring older adult-led health promotion must systematically integrate older adults into the fabric of the organization and not relegate them to select areas of programming. This entails a flexible way of viewing potential older adult contributions to the organization and community, including leadership.

7. The goals of older adult-led health promotion are best addressed through active and meaningful collaboration between consumers, providers, community, and academics. These partnerships should

always be led by older adults, with appropriate and requested support on their part. Goals related to older adult health promotion go beyond narrow definitions of what constitutes health, and therefore require broad and encompassing representation in health promotion interventions.

8. Definitions of health in health promotion are not universal and, as a consequence, must be shaped by the sociocultural values and beliefs of the intended recipients of the intervention, namely, older adults themselves. This necessitates that time and effort be prioritized to the development of a definition of health that is centered on how older adults define health. Age is but one factor that will enter into this definition. Other factors, such as gender, sexual identity, ethnicity/race, socioeconomic status, and religious beliefs, to mention but a few, are also part of how health is defined.

9. Active efforts to disseminate the results and findings of older adult-led health promotion should represent one of the goals of this type of intervention. This is an unusual principle, and it does not mean that dissemination must be exclusively "scholarly" in nature. Presentations by older adults to older adult–serving organizations, other older adults, newspaper articles, and organizational newsletter articles, for example, represent important forms of dissemination.

10. As touched upon in principle 4, older adult-led health promotion must not be narrowly defined to reach only older adults. This form of health promotion can also be conceptualized to reach audiences across the entire life cycle, as well as lending itself to intergenerational efforts. Older adult-led health promotion, similar to youth-led health promotion, must benefit more than the age group leading the effort; although specific age groups can be the primary beneficiaries of the intervention, they are certainly not the only beneficiaries.

SELF-CARE

There are certainly numerous points of view on how to bring older adult health promotion to life. Self-care has emerged as a multidimensional construct with important implications for how to conceptualize older adult-led health promotion and how to target people of color across the life span. However, its value is further increased when discussing older adults of color in urban contexts, since the role of cultural belief systems and past experiences with formal health care may shape their views of health care for themselves and their families.

Self-care has emerged as a critical element in older adult-led health promotion from both an assessment and a programming perspective. It is important to emphasize, however, that self-care is much more than an individual's response to symptoms, since it also entails the representation and interpretation of self (Dill, Brown, Clambrone, & Rakowski, 1990). McDonald-Miszczak, Wister, and Gutman (2001), for example, examined self-care among older adults from the perspective of their behaviors involving arthritis and conclude that objective factors and illness-specific beliefs are better predictors of health behavior when compared to illnesses, such as heart problems and hypertension, which tend to draw upon general beliefs.

The representation and interpretation of self increases in prominence among older adults of color because of their long history in undertaking self-care due to a reluctance to trust health care systems that have historically discriminated against them, resulting in disparate care of low quality. Self-efficacy, as already noted in the preceding chapter, is also closely tied to self-care beliefs and practices. This close association lends itself quite well for incorporation into older adult health promotion strategies.

My interest in self-care and health can be traced back to the mid-1970s as a result of research and scholarship on Latino folk healing (Delgado, 1977, 1979). It became quite evident to me that Latino older adults were the primary providers of self-care knowledge and practice within the Latino community in the United States, and this knowledge and practice could be traced back centuries and were an integral part of the culture (Delgado, 1995, 2007). I found self-care knowledge and practices to be well integrated within cultural traditions and beliefs, affirming and representing indigenous efforts to address health care needs within the community, and as a counter to a health care system that was at best unresponsive and at worst deadly.

Becker and colleagues' (2004, p. 2067) observations pertaining to African Americans can also be made for other groups of color such as Latinos, Native Americans, and Asian and Pacific Islanders: "African Americans have a long tradition of health and healing practices that shape, in part, what they do to care for themselves in the present day. African Americans' traditional medicine can be traced back beyond enslavement in the United States to their native cultures in Africa." The authors' conclusions touch upon the integral nature of self-care and culture and their importance in the lives of older adults of color and their communities. Older adult health promotion, as a result, must assess the nature and extent of self-care, and attempt to incorporate where possible the values and beliefs accordingly.

Marks and Allegrante (2005) stress the importance and role of self-efficacy enhancing health promotion practice. Fuzhong, Fisher, Harmer, and McAuley (2005) examined self-efficacy as a mediator of older adult (seventy to ninety-two years of age) fears of falling during tai chi exercising. The results showed the importance of health promotion initiatives designed to improve fall self-efficacy as an integral part of an exercise intervention. Easom (2003), too, stresses the role of perceived self-efficacy as a facilitating and hindering factor in self-care activities.

SOCIAL AND ECONOMIC JUSTICE AND EMPOWERMENT

As already noted in chapter 3, it is artificial to disassociate or divorce civic engagement from the social reality of older adults, and Marks and Shive (2007) bring this very point to the fore:

> In the present-day heterogeneous world, as well as in the United States where wide disparities in health and social conditions continue to exist, achievements in health are not uniform for all. Because of the pervasive and continuous impact of poverty on health and the prevailing economic and educational inequalities that flow from this, a concerted effort is needed to prevent widening or stagnant health inequalities, despite commendable progress in many areas of the United States (p. 30).

Older adults who are marginalized because of social characteristics, circumstances, or belief systems view their immediate world, life, and health through that lens (Angel & Angel, 2006). Conversely, older adults with privileged backgrounds, too, will engender civic engagement through their experiences and worldview. The former may view volunteering as a privilege; the latter may view it as a right. Priorities for engagement, as a consequence, will be shaped accordingly. This necessitates viewing older adult-led health promotion through a social and economic justice lens because of how this book has focused on urban older adults of color and the role of empowerment as a vehicle for achieving this goal.

The emergence of a social determinant of health perspective in the field of health promotion, along with a wider corresponding acceptance of an ecological viewpoint that places the health of individuals within a broader social context, necessitates an articulation of how values determine how health within context is viewed. Seeman (2000), in a study of health-promoting effects of family and friends on health outcomes of older adults, found further evidence of why an ecological perspective, in this case social network–focused, has a valuable place in any conceptualization of older adult health promotion practice. The clearer these values are promulgated, the easier it becomes for the field to accept or debate their presence and scope. This chapter grounds older adult-led health promotion, particularly in the case of urban older adults of color, within a social and economic justice value stance. As noted earlier in this book, social and economic justice values guide how health is defined and considered and how health promotion initiatives are guided.

The reader may initially react with puzzlement as to why the subject of social and economic justice enters into a book on health promotion and older adults. However, not addressing this very critical point in an open manner would effectively limit the potential of health promotion with this population group, particularly when discussing socially and economically marginalized older adults of color in this society. All social interventions, regardless of their nature and the target group, are based upon a set of values and principles. Sometimes they are explicit; other times, they are implicit. The more explicit they become, the easier it is to analyze and comment upon them. Older adult-led health promotion is no exception to this line of reasoning.

Health promotion and older adults can be guided through the use of a variety of principles, as already addressed earlier in this chapter. This guidance, so to speak, seeks to aid practitioners and academics alike in better conceptualizing and implementing health promotion strategies with this age group. A significant number of scholars in the fields of public health and social work, for example, have effectively argued for a health promotion agenda that is deeply rooted within a social and economic justice foundation, as a means of fighting against ageism and a number of other forms of social oppression. Grounding health and health promotion within such a context will naturally lead to efforts to better understand and address social determinants of health. Chapin and Cox (2001), for example, have argued that a shift in paradigms from deficits to strengths and empowerment are natural connections that will serve all older adults well, particularly those who are frail, and one can add, low-wealth/low-income older adults of color. The perspective that emerges through the use of a social and economic justice lens grounds consumer-led health promotion with older adults within a value base that stresses equality of opportunity, regardless of the sociodemographic background. This universal quality is quite attractive because it strives to acknowledge discriminatory experiences that these older adults have had in their lifetime. However, it takes on even greater appeal when the older adult group being targeted is severely marginalized or undervalued in this society because of some set of social factors such as gender, socioeconomic status, sexual identity, or race and ethnicity. Some academics or practitioners may argue that this "politicizes" health. However, it would be naïve to think that "politics," or social context, if you wish, does not influence how health is conceptualized and treated in all sectors of this country.

The concept of social and economic justice, simply referred to as social justice, is one that can be found in virtually any helping profession's credo or mission statement and code of ethics. This concept has found particular viability when used to describe social interventions targeting marginalized or undervalued groups in this country. These groups, as a result of an interplay of social factors such as race, gender, abilities, sexual orientation, and socioeconomic class, find their existence compromised in this society. This compromised state translates into some form of disparity—in the case of this book, health related.

Readers can rightly question whether older adults in this society fall into an undervalued category. For the most part, older adults have access to health and income, are a powerful voting constituency, and in the eyes of many, are a "privileged" age group. However, when examining particular subgroups, this so-called "privileged" state quickly disappears, exposing certain groups of older adults to a wide range of social challenges, including access to quality health care, as noted in chapter 4. Limited health care options increase the health risks of older adults (Burgener, 2004).

Ageism is probably the most popular construct used to describe social issues related to social and economic justice and older adults (Cameron, 2006). Wilson, Steele, Simson, and Harlow-Rosentraub (2006) note that terms such as *grey peril*, *greedy geezers*, and *the hippopotamus in the living room*, typify the prevalence of national concerns and fears about how the increasing number of older adults will use more than their share of natural resources. None of these terms seek to empower older adults in their quest to achieve health and well-being. In fact, they seek to achieve the opposite goal of disempowering them by making them feel shame for achieving the status of old age.

EMPOWERMENT AS A HEALTH PROMOTION VEHICLE

Empowerment is a critical component of most health promotion models, and this is particularly the case in any consumer-led health promotion effort such as the one advocated in this book. Squire (2001), in a succinct review of the literature on empowerment and older adults, concludes that empowerment is a central ideology and practice of health promotion, and that it must extend beyond the individual older adult to also encompass their family and community. Romero (1999), as cited in Story (2007), identifies a series of strategies for recognizing the main tenets of empowerment that have applicability to older adults, such as increasing knowledge base, identifying interpersonal, cultural, social, and economic barriers, developing competencies, and developing a plan of action.

As noted in chapter 1, older adult-led health promotion is best appreciated and understood within the broader context of consumer-led health
care in the national and international arenas (Lette, 2003; Nelson-Lye,
2007; Tomes, 2006). Nelson-Lye (2007) rightly equates consumer-led
health care with consumer empowerment:

> Consumer empowerment within health has sought to empower patients
> with the right and ability to maintain their health by "doing their home
> work" and becoming more knowledgeable as well as becoming more ac-
> tively engaged in managing their health care and making better health care
> decisions. This process as such has required health care providers to become
> more transparent, more ethical, with a greater degree of quality assurance,
> advocacy and inclusivity (p. 6).

Young and colleagues (2005) conclude that consumer-led interventions
serve to improve provider competencies in domains that are necessary
for high-quality care. Advocates of the consumer-led health movement
stress the important role consumers can play in educating providers to
better understand and address health care from a cultural and linguistic
perspective (Multicultural Mental Health Australia, 2003). Consumer-led
health promotion is a movement that is not bound by national boundaries, age groups, or health topics, and effectively serves to ensure that
services reflect the priorities and perspectives of consumers.

Older adults face a unique set of social circumstances that effectively
result in a loss of power and influence, with the loss of independence
and privacy being two of the greatest losses (Mahoney & Zooda, 2006).
Minkler (2000, p. 355), too, notes that the field's embrace of concepts
such as community empowerment and participation reflect a commitment to such precepts as the common good and shared responsibility
for health: "Acting on these concepts means enabling communities to
participate, in equal partnership with health professionals, in setting the
health agenda defining their health problems and helping to develop
the solutions to address those problems." Such a perspective on health
promotion, incidentally, fits well with definitions of health that are culturally grounded, as often found in many African American, Asian, and
Latino communities. Values of interdependence, for example, bring a
broader view of the "social good," and in the process are also culturally
complementary.

The social context that older adults operate within is of critical importance in determining how they view their health and the options that they
have to exercise control over it. A community that is disempowered, as
a result, will make it arduous for the older adult to become empowered.
Empowerment of older adults must occur concomitantly with empowerment of community. The emphasis placed on consumer empowerment

in consumer-led health care, for example, translates quite well to older adult-led health promotion and to increasing older adult participation in the decision-making process surrounding their health and the health of their respective communities.

The concept of empowerment has enjoyed tremendous popularity the past twenty years and, not surprisingly, has also enjoyed a wide range of definitions. The emergence and universal appeal of empowerment has been extraordinary. However, it is a concept that remains quite arduous to define, even after all of these decades, since it emerged in the professional literature. Empowerment is probably best defined as a vision for self-improvement and self-determination (Fetterman, 2003). There are a multitude of perspectives on empowerment, such as a philosophical stance, a goal, a process, and an outcome. Consequently, this multifaceted perspective further clouds what is meant by empowerment and how it becomes operational in the research and practice arenas.

The reader can no doubt discern that the definition of empowerment provided here has a number of primary goals imbedded within. Empowerment has three primary goals:

1. increase capacity to achieve change (individual, group, and community levels)—process objective
2. achievement of specific outcomes in shaping the environment—output objective
3. creation of group and community leadership and shared community collective experiences that can be mobilized to address other social and economic injustices—impact objective

When empowerment is viewed from this multilevel perspective, it is not unique to any one sociodemographic group, and it can be considered universal in appeal and applicability. Nevertheless, it takes on added appeal and significance in situations where the individual and their community have long histories of being disempowered and not having their voices heard by people in authority.

Empowerment can occur in a variety of settings and ways. Tjia, Givens, Karlawish, Okoli-Umeweni, & Barg (2007), for example, recommend greater use of educational messages promoting patient-physician dialogue to increase older adult shared decision making with physicians in type 2 diabetes treatment. However, their recommendations have implications that go far beyond this disease. It would be unreasonable to expect older adults, particularly those with histories of not having been encouraged to share their opinions on their health care, to simply and effortlessly enter into patient-initiated dialogue or shared decision making with physicians. An educational campaign that stresses shared decision making can be an initial step in bringing about a greater role in health care delivery for older adults. This can be accomplished in a variety of ways. However, the showing of a video in multiple languages modeling a patient-physician interaction that stresses decision making can be shown in a waiting room, for example.

Raeburn and Corbett (2001, p. 3) comment on the attractiveness of community development for promoting community health: "Nowhere are the issues more dramatically represented in the domain of community development as applied to HP. For us, and for many, community development and its cousin empowerment, represent the true heartland of HP. And at the heart of CD and HP . . . is the concept of 'people-centredness.'" C. D. Austin, DesCamp, Flux, McCleland, and Sleppert (2005), however, argue that although community practice has a relatively long history in social work, it has been overlooked regarding older adults, and it is time that this method of intervention be used by gerontological social workers. Such an approach effectively shifts the traditional focus in gerontology from disability and dependency to one that is empowerment and community-capacity-enhancement oriented.

The reader may well raise the important question, where does health promotion begin and end when placed within a community and community development context? The answer to this question is at the crux of community development and health promotion. The answer is not static, making a consensus on the "boundaries" of health promotion arduous and, some would argue, impossible to make. Nevertheless, a challenge such as this will not prevent the development of community-focused initiatives, even though they may be challenged by critics and will be arduous to evaluate (Moxley & Hyduk, 2003).

The construct of empowerment has found its way into the gerontological field into such diverse areas as

1. women (Browne, 1995; Narushima, 2004)
2. the frail (Huemann, McCall, & Boldy, 2001)
3. the incarcerated or institutionalized (Delgado & Humm-Delgado, 2008)
4. LGBT (Domahue & McDonald, 2005)
5. evaluation (Hurworth, Harvey, & Rutter, 2002)
6. spirituality (King, et al., 2005)
7. HIV/AIDS (Poindexter, 2004; Poindexter & Krigher, 2004)
8. alternative therapies (Arcury, Bell, Vitolinas, & Quandt, 2005)
9. strength training (Katula, Sipe, Rejeski, & Focht, 2006)
10. education (Ginsberg, 2001)
11. diabetes self-care (DeCoster & George, 2005), and
12. health promotion (Wieck, 2000)

As the reader can no doubt discern from this list, there is virtually no area where empowerment cannot or should not play a prominent role with older adults as a central focus.

A number of other constructs can find a place within empowerment. Thus, empowerment becomes an "umbrella" in similar fashion to community capacity enhancement. For example, according to Chapin and Cox (2001), empowerment and strength-based practice share certain basic assumptions and place older adults in a central role in shaping and carrying out interventions. Bullock and McGraw (2006), in a project focused on breast and cervical cancer screening among older women of color, too, stress the importance of enhancing informal support networks in the process of conducting screening. Active participation (empowerment) in the decision-making process is often the hallmark of capacity enhancement practice at the individual, group, and community levels (Delgado, 2000).

Assertiveness training for older adults, for example, has been recommended as a means of empowering them to fight against age discrimination (Vann, 2006). This form of training, however, has generally not been offered to older adults. Supporting older adults in assessing their circumstances and situation, evaluating their feelings and needs, and planning appropriate actions are all transferable skills. However, these skills take on greater significance in the case of older adults of color who must fight not only age discrimination but racial discrimination as well.

McWilliam and colleagues (1997), in a study specifically focused on empowerment and health promotion and chronically ill older adults, identify five health-promoting strategies for creating empowering meaning for this group of elders: (1) building trust and meaning, (2) connecting, (3) caring, (4) mutual knowing, and (5) mutual creating. Each of these elements or dimensions, in turn, seeks to tap an aspect of older adults' lives that is affirming of their experiences and potential, as well as setting the necessary groundwork for action, as in the case of older adult-led health promotion. Some of these elements were addressed specifically to a subgroup of older adults; their applicability to other older adults, such as low-income/low-wealth older adults of color, is quite strong.

OLDER ADULT HEALTH PROMOTERS AS QUASI-VOLUNTEERS AND STAFF

The field may raise questions or even concerns about changing what is meant by civic engagement. Is civic engagement synonymous with volunteering, or are we talking about a totally new role, particularly in the case of low-income/low-wealth older adults as health promoters? There is no denying the need for low-income/low-wealth older adults to earn an income to help offset the costs associated with volunteering. Consequently, concepts are expected to be dynamic in quality to be able to adapt to changing circumstances. Civic engagement, as a result, is not immune from these forces, as noted in chapter 3.

Economic incentives, such as scholarships for children or grandchildren of their choosing, reduced costs for prescriptions, stipends, and special discounts for local purchases and entertainment, are often found to be significant motivators to get older adults to volunteer, especially when they have limited financial means (Saint Paul Foundation, 2007). Providing economic incentives in no way diminishes the volunteering experience. In fact, it enhances it. Volunteerism resulting from economic incentives represents a serious attempt to value the "wealth" and importance of their contributions. Older adults as health promotion consultants and project advisors, for example, have been reported in the literature (Haber & Looney, 2003).

Civic engagement involving low-income/low-wealth older adults, as a result, must be broadened to include participation that historically would not "qualify" as volunteerism. This is particularly important in the case of older adult women who, because of histories of pay inequality, have smaller retirement savings compared with their male counterparts (Hawthorne, 2007).

The emergence of the concept of "paid volunteerism" helps to capture both the spirit of volunteerism as well as the reality of older adults with low-income/low-wealth backgrounds receiving monetary compensation for their efforts. The *New York Times* recently published an article titled "For Love and a Little Money," addressing a new status called paid volunteerism (Deutsch, 2007). The benefits of receiving compensation for "volunteering" go beyond payment, since there is the added bonus of having the work appreciated by the host organization. Paid volunteers receive monetary compensation that is significantly lower than the market rate for comparable services.

OLDER ADULT HEALTH PROMOTION FRAMEWORK

The relationship between theoria (knowledge) and praxis (action) is quite close, with each relying upon the other to maintain relevance in social interventions, and with frameworks being the "glue" or "connector" between these two concepts. Glanz, Lewis, and Rimer (1997), in discussing health education and promotion, rightly note that theory and research are not the exclusive domains of academia, and practice is not solely the domain of professional practitioners. Consumers of health promotion, too, need to weigh into the theory and practice equation! Frameworks not only help theoreticians and practitioners, but they also assist consumers in their participation in health promotion initiatives. In essence, use of frameworks is a win-win for all of the different parties that are involved in health promotion.

Analytical frameworks help gather data and dictate interventions and should be thought of as a tool to assist in the building of a program or project. Practitioners, consumers, and academics need a tool that can help them place health promotion efforts within a constellation of programs and projects that can be found in the field and literature. Like any tool, however, it is only as good as the individual's skill that is using it. In the hands of a skilled person, it is wonderful; in the hands of an unskilled practitioner, it is useless. The framework on older adult health promotion that follows only represents one of countless different ways of conceptualizing the field and its incorporations, or lack thereof depending upon where on the framework one focuses, of older adults in the planning, implementation, and evaluation of programs. The youth development/youth-led field, for example, has its share of "continuums" and "frameworks" that play important roles in helping to create a better understanding and shaping of interventions focused on youth. However, the older adult field has not benefited from this type of attention.

The reader may take issue with how I have characterized the various viewpoints and stages. The field can certainly entertain other frameworks, particularly those that are empowering of older adults and their communities. The following continuum represents an initial attempt at better understanding the role and importance of older adults in shaping health promotion efforts that target them.

Table 6.1 provides a visual representation of seven ways of viewing or categorizing health promotion and older adults. Each of these stages or steps represents both a view of older adults and a role they can play in a health promotion project. At one end of the framework (*service-focus*), they play the conventional role as consumers, and the health promoter (professional) is the ultimate decision maker. This is a very traditional perspective that can also be called deficit driven. At the opposite end of the framework (*older adult-led*) is the most progressive, or radical, view of older adult health promotion, which places them in the ultimate position of power and is community-capacity-enhancement driven.

The framework presented in table 6.1 helps organizations sponsoring older adult health promotion to conceptualize organizational values pertaining to empowerment of older adults, community-capacity enhancement, and their interventions involving partnerships with the community. As the reader has no doubt noticed, each stage of this framework can be viewed from one of six perspectives, ending in how evaluation gets conceptualized and carried by older adults. Organizational movement

Table 6.1. Framework for Older Adult Health Promotion

Health Promotion Project Facet	Stage 1 Service Focus	Stage 2 Development Focused	Stage 3 Leadership Focused	Stage 4 Civic Engagement	Stage 5 Engagement with Staff Support	Stage 6 Engagement with Staff Consultation	Stage 7 Older-Led
Primary Goal	Individual Disease/ Illness Treatment	Individual Treatment & Capacity Enhancement	Individual Capacity Enhancement	Individual Capacity Enhancement	Individual Capacity Enhancement	Community Capacity Enhancement	Community Capacity Enhancement
Focus of Promotion	Individual	Individual	Individual	Individual	Individual	Individual	Community
Process Driven	Staff Driven	Staff Driven	Staff Driven	Staff Driven	Older Adult Driven w/ Staff Support	Older Adult Driven w/ Staff Support	Older Adult & Community Driven
Target of Promotion	Individual	Individual	Individual	Individual	Individual	Individual	Community
Setting Focus	Agency Based	Agency Based	Agency Based	Agency/ Community Base	External Agency & Community Based	External Agency & Community Based	Community Based
Evaluation	Staff Driven	Staff Driven	Staff Driven	Staff Driven	Staff Driven with Older Adult Input	Older Adult Driven with Staff Input	Community Driven

across the framework can probably best be viewed developmentally, though cases where organizations started out at the two farthest ends of the framework no doubt exist. It is safe to say, however, that most organizations sponsoring older adult health promotion efforts are not at the most progressive end of the continuum, unfortunately.

How best to conceptualize and categorize health promotion and older adult efforts is a constant challenge in the field, not dissimilar from efforts involving other age groups such as youth (Delgado & Zhou, 2008). The following brief description of all of the stages covered in table 6.1 provides the reader with more details than those provided in the table.

1. **Older Adult Services Focused**: This stage is characterized by the conventional view of older adults as consumers or clients. Older adults, as a result, do not wield decision-making powers over the programs and projects that target them. In addition, they are not generally viewed as possessing strengths or considered as assets in the community. In essence, older adults are in need of having their health promoted and are expected to be passive consumers because they are not the experts of their own health. This stage is without question the most disempowering stage in the framework because it makes older adults passive recipients of health services.

2. **Older Adult Development Approach**: This stage is characterized by seeking to build on older adult competencies and making them more independent on health matters. The emphasis of this stage, however, still remains very much on service provision (health education) versus development or enhancement, although there is a reluctant acknowledgment that older adults do possess strengths that can be mobilized in service to themselves—but not their communities. This stage, as a result, takes a very a narrow view of older adult strengths and who can benefit from them, and still places professional providers in the position of being the experts on older adult health.

3. **Older Adult Leadership**: This stage provides older adults with opportunities to assume limited leadership roles within organizations and projects because it explicitly acknowledges their assets and potential for positive contributions to the organization and the community. This stage, however, is still individual older adult focused, rather than reflecting a programmatic or mission-driven agenda to systematically involve older adults in leadership positions. Thus, this stage is dependent upon the "exceptional" older adult, rather than a concerted effort to move older adults into leadership positions. As already noted, there is an acknowledgment that older adults have assets and can play leadership roles within a circumspect arena, and

organizations are prepared to explore older adult civic engagement in this manner.

4. **Older Adult Civic Engagement**: Stage four encourages and provides opportunities for older adults to assume high profile leadership positions within organizations and communities. Decisions on who participates and the nature of the roles assumed are determined on a case-by-case approach. Nevertheless, unlike the previous stage, this stage reflects a programmatic thrust based upon a mission of the organization sponsoring the health promotion project. Structural mechanisms, in turn, are in place to provide necessary training and staff support that is required for older adults to make important and sustained contributions. These resources are viewed as an investment in social capital development and enhancement.

5. **Older Adult Engagement with Active Staff Support**: Stage five places older adults in key decision-making roles with active staff support to assist them throughout the entire process, and represents the continuation of an empowering perspective. The organization sponsoring older adult–focused health promotion projects sees meaningful older adult engagement as central to their mission and the health of the community, and as a result, is prepared to provide meaningful staff support and any other resources that are needed. There is a systematic assessment of the skill and knowledge sets that older adults possess. This action is critical in order for organizations to be strategic in their actions involving older adults. This assessment is built into how the organization recruits, screens, and provides support for older adults.

6. **Older Adult Engagement with Consultation as Needed**: Unlike stage five, this stage envisions older adults playing key decision-making roles but involves staff in consultative roles as needed and recommended. The mission guiding older adult health promotion efforts requires older adult leadership. Organizational support, in turn, can be manifested through a variety of mechanisms, one of which is having staff act as consultants on an as-needed basis to be determined by older adults. However, older adults may request other forms of support in order to carry out their mission to enhance the health of older adults and/or other community members. Attendance at workshops and conferences, for example, to enhance competencies in various areas may be requested and facilitated by host organizations. Field visits to organizations utilizing older adults in key decision-making roles may also be requested.

7. **Older Adult-Led Health Promotion**: This stage conceptualizes older adults as carrying out all of the key decision-making roles in the creation and implementation of projects. This form of older adult

engagement is the most significant and empowering in older adult health promotion. Organizational supports can be available when requested and can take on any form that older adults request. Stage seven can be considered the most progressive and empowering of all of the stages in this framework and can be an organizational goal that sponsoring entities strive to achieve.

The seven stages of older adult health promotion presented above provide the older adult health promotion field with a tool that helps categorize efforts and identify potential goals for organizations to strive for in the course of engaging and serving this population group. In review, the continuum presented in table 6.1 consists of seven stages that can be conceptualized from an empowerment perspective. Each progressive stage increases the degree of influence that older adults exercise in conceptualizing and implementing health promotion projects. The first stage (Older Adult Services Approach) is the least empowering, and the last stage (Older Adult-Led Health promotion) is the most empowering. Each of these stages, in turn, comes with the requisite analytical and interactional forces and considerations.

The slow but increased attention paid to older adults in this country has taken a variety of manifestations, with health promotion targeting this age group being but one example (Resnick, 2001a). Rabiner (2005) provides a conceptual framework for assessing the determinants and consequences of engaging older adults in health promotion interventions. This framework takes into account a variety of individual as well as community-wide outcomes. Most of the literature concerning older adult health in a social network of family and friends has viewed the health-promoting effects on older adults (Seeman, 2000). However, it is rare to see the reverse, namely, the effects of health promoting that older adults have on family, friends, and their respective communities.

OLDER ADULTS AS COMMUNITY AND HEALTH PROMOTION ASSETS

Older adults, particularly those who are marginalized because of income, race/ethnicity, gender, and abilities, have managed to live long lives. Their abilities to socially navigate their way through society's barriers should never be underestimated by policy makers, academics, and funders. Interestingly, cumulative psychosocial risks have received greater attention than cumulative resilience (Myers & Hwang, 2004). The concept of resilience, after all, is not age-restricted to youth and young adults. Yet it is rarely discussed from an older adult perspective. The American

Psychological Association (2004) has specifically issued a paper with the goal of fostering resilience on the part of older adults. In this instance, it is response to terrorism. This is an important area based upon the times that we live in. However, there is a need to broaden our perspective of how resiliency gets manifested and fostered in older adults.

Older adults of color in low-wealth/low-income circumstances have "survived" to get to this age. Consequently, much more research and attention needs to be placed on how they got so resilient rather than focusing on their health issues and social circumstances. Mind you, this perspective on resiliency does not mean that older adults do not suffer from various illnesses and diseases, as already noted in great detail in chapter 4 and elsewhere throughout this book. It does mean, however, that prior to examining health needs, it is necessary to start with their assets as a background to better understanding needs.

Is the glass half full or half empty? The reader may look at this question and say it is all semantics. I do beg to differ, however. A resiliency-/assets-first perspective effectively broadens the horizon of what information is important. An assets-first perspective influences the terms and vocabulary that older adults use to characterize their life circumstances and situations, and dramatically alters any conversation regarding older adults and health.

Society has been slow in shifting a prevailing view of older adults as not possessing strengths or assets. Showkeir (1974), well over thirty-five years ago and in probably one of the earliest scholarly articles on older adults as community assets, argued for society to shift its views toward older adults. The American Society on Aging (2007, p. 2) makes a similar argument for this shift: "While more and more adults are experiencing longer periods of healthy retirement, our society still predominantly sees old age as a time of problems and time of letting go: of jobs, friends, strenuous recreation, and life itself. Whether that age does bring loss, less recognized is the potential of elders to lead full contributive lives." Experiencing losses or changes does not automatically translate into not having strengths or assets. Life, after all, is never one or the other. No other age group suffers from such a one-sided perspective, and why should older adults?

Freedman (1999) traces the emergence of older adults as an "incurable disease," or deficit perspective, to the later part of the nineteenth century and the influence of human service professionals:

The new purveyors of antiaging nostrums were not evangelists but an emerging group of professionals—social workers, sociologists, management experts, and, most significantly, physicians—who positioned themselves as authorities on aging. Incapable of arresting or treating age-related maladies, these frustrated medicine men belittled the older generation and character-ized aging as an incurable, ever-worsening disease. No longer were the elderly seen as simply as older versions of younger people (p. 42).

Aging is a natural process rather than a diseased process with all of the connotations associated with this negative perspective.

A review of the literature on older adults as possessing strengths or assets will uncover a number of articles on the subject dating back to the mid-1980s (Gallagher, 1985; Milligan, Maryland, Ziegler, & Ward, 1987). From a cultural perspective for many groups of color, if not all, there has been an understanding and appreciation of older adults as providing in-strumental, experiential, and informational services, as well as transmis-sion of cultural values and historical information that shape ethnic and racial identity from a positive perspective. Unfortunately, the concept of older adults as being community assets and possessing strengths did not receive the attention that it warranted in both scholarly and funding circles. Fortunately, communities of color did not read or subscribe to this literature! All older adults, regardless of their present circumstances and level of functioning, have the potential to contribute. They have abilities and potential to contribute to their families, community, and society. Health promotion, particularly one that is led by the older adult him- or herself, must provide an affirming and empowering avenue for them to contribute (O'Neill, 2002).

There is still much to be learned about what factors motivate older adults to participate in healthy behaviors, particularly those persons who are not of the dominant culture (Miller & Iris, 2002, p. 250): "Therefore, the key to identifying appropriate markers of successful health promo-tion is to ascertain the components of health and well-being that are most relevant and meaningful to older adults. It is equally important to elucidate strategies and motivating factors that are most likely to impel older people to participate in such programs. This implies use of an emic approach which explores meanings, values, and goals from the perspec-tives of older adults themselves."

Cleak and Howe's (2003) study of social networks and use of social supports of older adults of color in East Harlem (New York City) found that the importance of urban social networks in health and well-being cannot be underestimated, particularly in the use of informal support. Locher and colleagues (2004) found that social isolation plays an impor-tant role in increasing nutritional risk, and they stress the importance of creating active social networks as part of health promotion interventions. Greenwald and Beery (2001) found it possible to design interventions to reduce older adult isolation. Buijs, Ross-Kerr, O'Brien, and Wilson (2003), in a Canadian study of health promotion participation on the part of older adults with low incomes, conclude that fun, program flexibility, autonomy, social interactions among participations and staff-participant relationships all played critical roles in participants developing a sense of comfort with the program and increasing participation. Thus, the benefits derived from socialization and social support can be a powerful motivator for participation. Assessment, as a result, becomes an important step in older adult-led health promotion. This assessment, however, must involve both assets as well as a multifaceted (social, physical, and emotional) perspective on the needs of older adults.

OLDER ADULT-LED HEALTH PROMOTION

As already initially addressed in chapter 1, older adult leadership and active involvement in shaping and delivering health promotion services is certainly not a new concept in the field (Ho et al., 1987; Lynde, 1992; Sutherland et al., 1988; Weinrich et al., 1993). However, older adult-led health promotion, with all of the symbols and consequences associated with this paradigm, is relatively new in the fields of health promotion and gerontology, although its legacy can be traced back several decades.

Gordon (2004, p. 28) notes that "health promotion is often portrayed as a matter of individual responsibility and personal choice. But access to culturally appropriate programs and facilities must exist for the projected 20,000,000 older adults of color to embrace personal responsibility and enjoy good health promotion choices." When choices are severely limited, the option of exercising choice is an illusion. One size of health promotion, older adult-led or the more conventional type, is not what the field needs to be relevant in the lives of all older adults and not just the privileged. Further, the field is in need of new roles for older adults that are enriching for them and benefit the community in general, and not just other older adults.

Miller and Iris (2002) identify the need for health promotion programs attempting to reach older adults to provide socialization and social support as central features in encouraging participation. The importance of social relationships is often mentioned in the literature as a key motivator for engaging older adults of color. Health promotion programs must, as a result, also provide flexibility in choice of activities and structures to increase participant sense of control over their participation. The issue of "control" over the goals, nature, and extent of participation in health programs becomes prominent when the target group consists of older adults, although the same considerations should apply to all groups.

Tension between health promoters and consumers can manifest itself in a variety of ways, with degree of older adult participation being but one of the critical measures. Older adult-led health promotion shifts control from professionals to consumers and, in the process of doing so, necessitates professionals' reconceptualizing their roles to ones of facilitators and consultants, as opposed to managers, coordinators, and supervisors. This shift, incidentally, is easier said than done because very few professional education programs prepare professionals to assume roles as supporters of health promotion programs, as opposed to designers and decision makers. Further, such a shift in roles requires considerable scholarship and research to provide the requisite documentation often required before a novel idea eventually works its way into a curriculum.

RECRUITMENT OF OLDER ADULT HEALTH PROMOTERS

Finding community settings for recruitment and training of older adults to conduct health promotion represents one of the initial and, some would argue, one of the biggest challenges facing the field of health promotion. Locating and gaining the support and legitimacy of community settings often represents the initial and, arguably, the most challenging step in older adult-led health promotion. Consequently, the finding of settings within a community that have a large cadre of older adult volunteers, and an atmosphere conducive for volunteering, is the most logical first step in recruiting older adult health promoters.

Since houses of worship are probably the most common places for volunteer activities among older adults, these settings represent ideal places for older adult-led health promotion initiatives to transpire, and as a possible resource for older adult health promoters. Older adult health promoters are in the advantageous position of knowing their congregations and enjoying their trust. Further, they will probably be most comfortable in these settings. This does not mean, however, that they cannot expand beyond that setting in conducting health promotion. Starting in these settings provides an excellent initial point to gain experience and confidence before moving out into the broader community and into new settings.

Health professionals gaining entry into houses of worship will present a series of challenges that must be addressed if the initiative or project is to succeed in a timely manner:

1. Religious leaders may be very suspicious of nonmember outsiders.
2. Health providers must be cognizant of the cultural values and be sufficiently bilingual to engage in dialogue in cases where English is not the primary language used by the congregation.

3. The process of engagement and commitment may be labor and time intensive since religious officials may not share the same time frames as professionals (grant deadlines, for example).
4. Providers must be prepared to enter into a form of dialogue that necessitates self-disclosure about their own definitions of God and religious practices.
5. Organizations sponsoring these types of initiatives must be prepared to be flexible with staff assigned to the roles as facilitators.
6. Data gathering pertaining to evaluation of initiatives must be modified to take into account the uniqueness of the setting.

The potential of houses of worship playing an influential role in older adult-led health promotion has been addressed earlier in this book, with numerous scholars singing the virtues of this setting for reaching older adults of color in a place where they feel comfortable and trusting. Nevertheless, the path toward fruitful health promotion collaboration is fraught with potential limitations and barriers, although the rewards are plentiful for the right sponsoring organization and staff. Organizational settings and staff with the commitment and capability of initiating health promotion efforts must also be prepared to assist others in exploring collaboration with houses of worship by acting as a bridge between these institutions and other formal health and social service organizations.

Community gatherings such as health fairs, health home parties, and health festivals provide both a place and space that is nonstigmatizing and celebratory, a place to both socialize and engage in health-promoting activities. These types of gatherings represent alternatives to houses of worship to both conduct health promotion and recruit older adults to deliver health promotion. Sadler and colleagues (2006), for example, strongly advocate the use of health parties as a viable recruitment strategy because it is a supportive and relatively inexpensive way to reach African Americans. These parties are sometimes referred to as "Tupperware parties without the sale" (National Cancer Institute, 2007). These types of gatherings provide ample opportunities to share health information, including where screenings can take place, as well as address fears participants may have that act as a barrier to health promotion participation. Most importantly, these events are held in people's homes and are therefore accessible geographically, psychologically, culturally, and operationally.

Resnick (2000b), in a study of health promotion focused on the old-old (ninety years or older), utilized a "Wellness Day" approach in a continuing care facility, and found that an individualized approach with each recipient proved the most effective method. An individualized focus has allowed health promoters an opportunity to connect with participants and tailor both their presentation efforts and follow-ups accordingly. A group approach, though less labor intensive, does not facilitate the relationship-building process and individualized attention often favored by older adults, old-old or otherwise. Old-old adults as a group have been found to be less likely than other older adult age groups to have their stools checked for occult blood, skin checked for lesions, or to have a recent mammogram, Pap test, or prostate examination (Resnick, 2003a). Consequently, this age group necessitates health promotion programs that take their unique circumstances into account when designing interventions (Resnick, 2000a, 2001b, 2003b,c). These types of activities can serve both as a strategy for delivering health promotion and recruitment of older adult health promoters.

OLDER ADULT-LED HEALTH PROMOTION ROLES

The broadness or expansiveness of the field of health promotion necessitates the creation of a wide variety of roles to carry out this form of intervention. Roles for older adults in older adult-led health promotion, for example, can consist of some or all of the following types: (1) advocate, (2) enabler or facilitator, (3) educator, (4) mediator, (5) researcher, (6) trainer, (7) administrative/logistical supporter. No one older adult is expected to carry out all of these roles or to do so with equal abilities and enthusiasm, just like no youth or adult would be expected to do so. Older adults are not super human beings who can assume any role at a drop of a hat. Each of these roles, in turn, requires different skill sets in order to achieve maximum results.

The question of the amount of time older adults devote to older adult-led health promotion efforts is bound to enter into any discussion of this type of experience, and the answer is very much determined by the role(s) they will undertake in the project and the organizational resources at their disposal. Time commitment to a project can consist of combinations until it becomes operational: (1) short but more intensive period of activity or (2) longer duration but shorter periods of intensity. Training, however, is generally outside of this time period. The amount of effort (time and resources) devoted to enhancing the skills and knowledge of older adults in health promotion will naturally vary according to local circumstances. Nevertheless, the resources invested in training and organizational support are critical to the overall success of any older adult-led health promotion project.

PROVIDER AS FACILITATOR

The emergence of new ways of thinking about older adult participation in leading health promotion efforts requires innovative ways of thinking about how this participation gets realized. The term *volunteer management practices* has been used to describe both the formal and informal approaches toward organizations and their professional staff working with volunteers. However, this term does not do justice to what will be needed on the part of staff and organizations to initiate and support older adult-led health promotion programs, such as the one this book is devoted to. The concept of "older adult led" is one that is rarely found in professional educational programs or even in professional conferences. Consequently, staff will have to learn as they go, so to speak.

Practitioners may wonder aloud about what role, if any, they have in older adult-led health promotion. The role of expert as facilitator provides professionals with an important role in helping consumers carry out health promotion initiatives. Hirschhorn (1979) almost thirty years ago advocated for the reconceptualization of provider-consumer relationships. This meant reconstituting conventional views of providers as experts and decision makers in the provision of services. A communal dialogue with facilitation serves as an educational, reflective, and empowering method for all participants in this inquiry (Kennedy, 2004).

Adlong (2006) places participatory inquiry into a facilitation/empowerment model. The shifting of power away from providers to consumers does not mean that providers cannot, and should not, play a meaningful role. It does mean, however, that consumers dictate the role and when it gets carried out. Being available to assist or facilitate is critical in consumer-led health promotion, older adult or youth-centered (Delgado & Zhou, 2008). Syme's (2000, p. 95) advice for the field of health promotion has profound implications for how we view our potential role in older adult-led health promotion: "The key lesson we health professionals should learn from the mistakes of the past is to be creative and inventive enough to become experts in the role of not being an expert." Older adults are the experts of their own lives and circumstances. We as professionals can best think of ourselves as collaborators with older adults.

Shifting from an expert to a collaborative role can be called many different terms. A "facilitative" or "reflective" role can also be called "participatory collaborative" (Sutton & Kemp, 2006). All of these terms and others not mentioned, however, capture an emerging perspective that is egalitarian in values, principles, and actions. The expert as facilitator is enjoying attention in the scholarly literature. Koch, Selim, and Kral (2002) specifically examined the health field and concluded that a facilitative or reflective process can enhance people's lives at both the individual and community level. Kakabadse and Kakabadse (2003) stress the importance of contextual relevance of experiential knowledge and the role providers can play in facilitating this discovery process. Fischer (2004) raises the role of expert as facilitator in the creation of meaningful social change. Mash and Meulenberg-Buskens (2001), in turn, note that facilitative or cooperative inquiry is a form of participatory action research for the development of health educational material and is relatively new but with tremendous potential for the field.

Adlong (2006) advances the use of a "collaborative inquiry group" as a vehicle for creating a context for both learning and working together to develop strategies for social action. These groups provide participants, in the case of this book, older adults, to construct "habits of thoughts" and form new collective ideas. "Respectful learning" fosters democratic interactions and creation of mutual trust, which are both conducive to the development of innovative solutions to local issues and priorities, such as older adult health. The group process and experience takes on greater significance than individual experiences, thereby reinforcing a sense of group and community connectedness.

In a literature review of barriers to older adult health education, four challenges were identified: (1) the decline in health literacy, (2) learning styles necessitating a multifaceted approach to conveying information, (3) belief systems (folk wisdom, traditions, spiritual practices, and customs), and (4) cultural barriers. Each of these barriers can exist in various manifestations, in combination with each other, and isolated, to make health education, and also health promotion, challenging for reaching older adults, particularly in the case of those who are not from the dominant culture (American Society on Aging, 2001). Lyle and Kasi (2002) highlight the educational gains of experts as facilitators for both consumers and providers. The process of "reflection" benefits all participating parties (Koch, Mann, Kralik, & van Loon, 2005). Tensions regarding the role as facilitator are not restricted to the provider-consumer relationship. Burgess (2006) provides a case example of how this tension can also be found in graduate school between student and professor.

Bandura and Schunk (1981) bring a complementary perspective that adds further depth to how staff can support older adults in their leading of health promotion efforts. The authors identified four primary sources of self-efficacy: (1) performance accomplishment, (2) vicarious experience, (3) verbal persuasion, and (4) emotional arousal. Health promotion staff must play instrumental roles in helping older adults, particularly those with histories of being marginalized and not having their voices heard, to increase their self-efficacy in order to undertake older adult-led health promotion. Although all four sources can be marshaled in service to this form of health promotion, verbal persuasion and emotional arousal are probably initially the two most important sources of support. Performance accomplishment and emotional arousal will naturally follow initial efforts at instituting projects.

Health promotion is far from being a monolithic strategy, as noted earlier in this chapter. Achieving health, as a result, lends itself to the use of a variety of concrete approaches that lend themselves to modifications that take into account local circumstances and goals to improve health and the conditions that cause illness. The complexity of health translates into the need for health promotion to adopt a multifaceted and, some would argue, complex approach that does justice to the importance of the topic.

Older adult-led health promotion brings a unique perspective to the fields of gerontology and health promotion, and in the process of doing so, also serves to bring other fields under its umbrella. Community social action and community development, for example, find a comfortable niche within this perspective as well. When social and economic justice and empowerment are front and center in steering this brand of health promotion, it seeks an inclusive rather than exclusive function.

Older adult-led health promotion is not static in conception, and as a result, holds much promise for helping to shape future models of this form of social intervention for older adults as well as other age and population groups. Consumer-led interventions have gathered momentum since the beginning of the millennium. Although these movements have taken particular shapes based upon the themes or constructs of the issues they address, they also share much in common when discussing marginalized groups; an ecological perspective helps connect these disparate fields.

7

New Arenas and Settings for Older Adult Health Promotion

"Over the past 10 years, 'settings' based health promotion has become a central figure of efforts to promote health that recognize the significance of context. Emerging in part from a perception of an over-reliance on individualistic methods, the approach was built on a profound belief in its value and deployed a range of novel theoretical resources. . . . This initial enthusiasm has been maintained within policy directives, in the professional literature and . . . amongst health promotion practitioners."

(Whitehead et al., 2001, p. 339)

The health promotion field has maintained its relevance and vibrancy through its creative approaches to how best to reach underserved population groups in this country, including the effective use of research findings in a timely manner. The process of putting into practice research findings is called "translational research." Translational research, according to the National Institutes of Health, "is the process of applying ideas, insights, and discoveries generated through basic scientific inquiry to the treatment and prevention of human disease."

Translation, in turn, is best conceptualized as consisting of two phases (Garfield et al., 2003, p. 2670): (1) "bench to bedside," or lab research to clinical research application; and (2) clinical research to "real-world" practice. However, each of these phases encounters potential barriers such as "behavioral impediments, cultural misunderstandings, poor diffusion of knowledge, underutilization of information technology, inefficient organization of care, financial disincentives, lack of insurance, and ineffective

149

public policies." Although these barriers to translational research apply
to a clinical setting, most of these barriers, with modifications, are also
applicable to health promotion.

Swerissen and Crisp (2004) apply the concept of sustainability to health
promotion and stress the need for the field to think creatively about what
is necessary to help ensure that successful interventions continue to receive funding. Jamner (2000, p. 7), in turn, challenges the field of health
promotion to embrace a desire to introduce innovations in exploring
potential new settings within which the field may be practiced: "In addition to mobilizing political will, another strategy with great potential for
enhancing the translation of scientific expertise into wellness promotion
is a greater reliance on nontraditional methods in both community and
clinical settings." Fortunately, this call for innovation is being heard in
the field as evidenced by the following two examples. Carson, Chappell,
and Knight (2007) report on the use of the arts within health promotion
programs as a means of reaching a wider community-based audience.
Cornisa and Ghosh (2006), in their study of a community-led health
promotion on HIV prevention in a red-light district of Calcutta, India,
also represent an innovative approach. This project reached out to sex
workers in men's clubs and brothels, health promotion settings that have
historically not been considered as part of conventional approaches to
HIV prevention. Panter-Brick and colleagues (2006), too, embrace a socioecological approach and report on the success of songs as a vehicle for
social change.

Health promotion settings are no longer viewed within a narrow interpretation, and as a result, new settings for health promotion have emerged
that contextualize this social intervention within a community (Baum,
2002). New ways of encouraging local development of health promotion
initiatives have also emerged that combine both health promotion and
community-capacity enhancement (Higgins, Naylor, & Day, 2008).

Health promotion and older adults, as a result, has benefited from innovative approaches and energy. As addressed in chapter 8, the development
of new research models and considerations to create a better understanding of the effectiveness of health promotion has also served to reinforce
this newfound attitude toward older adults and their health. This is an
attitude that can probably best be categorized as an emphasis on wellness,
disregarding the impact of illness and disease on their well-being.

Health promotion and older adults can be practiced in a wide variety
of settings that specifically focus on older adults. Health settings, senior
centers, and assisted living facilities, for example, have witnessed greater
attention as places where health promotion can be delivered. These are
certainly important settings based upon the high percentage of older
adults who make these places their home. However, there is a range of

informal settings, otherwise referred to as nontraditional settings, that also lends to health promotion initiatives (Delgado, 1999). These settings take on greater significance in the case of community- and urban-based older adults.

The following arenas or settings for health promotion typify the kind of thinking and creativity that will be needed for the field of health promotion to reach out to underserved older adult subgroups. Although there are countless urban community settings for health promotion to transpire, only four have been selected because of their importance and potential access for health promotion staff: (1) houses of worship, (2) beauty parlors and barbershops, (3) food establishments (restaurants, grocery stores, and bakeries), and (4) community gardens.

Each of these settings brings with it a set of rewards as well as challenges for the field of health promotion. Which of these settings is utilized is very much dependent upon local circumstances and the abilities and willingness (attitudes) of health promotion staff. Further, these types of settings are not monolithic in structure. The field, as a result, must be sufficiently flexible to take into account how local circumstances may shape each of these types of settings.

Houses of Worship

Religion and religiosity are subjects that the field of health promotion has historically understood the importance of and continues to do so as evidenced by the number of projects based in this setting. These projects, in turn, have addressed a wide variety of health concerns and have varied in the degree to which older adults have played instrumental roles in these types of interventions. Houses of worship provide important community settings that facilitate outreach to a number of underserved populations (Gelfand, 2003; Krause, 2004). This is particularly the case when discussing health promotion and African American and Latino urban communities across the country (Petterson, Atwood, & Yates, 2002). Cnaan, Boddie, and Kang (2005) argue that since a large proportion of older adults are affiliated with religious congregations, there is a built-in social care network that can be mobilized to provide a range of interventions such as social services and, we might add, health promotion. Religion and houses of worship represent, in essence, a largely untapped area for health promotion and communities of color.

The importance of religiosity is well recognized in the field, and not just around older adults. Duan, Fox, Derose, Carson, and Stockdale (2005) view houses of worship as possessing yet-unrealized great potential for provision of health education and the conducting of health-related research. Chen, Cheal, Herr, Zubritsky, and Levkoff (2007), in turn, conclude that religious participation is positively associated with older adults' mental health status and treatment effects. Religion among Latino and African-American older adults, for example, has been found to influence a wide range of attitudes and behaviors that clearly fall within an ecological view of health. This finding not only increases the number of possibilities for houses of worship to become partners in health promotion efforts, but it also brings with it a set of challenges for practitioners and academics alike.

However, research into the pathways that influence religious-health interconnectedness among African Americans still has a considerable distance to travel before there is widespread acceptance and recognition of the potential of these settings for conducting effective health promotion strategies (O'Neill, 2002; Sternberg, Munschauer, Carrow, & Sternberg, 2006). DeHaven, Hunter, Wilder, Walton, and Berry (2004), for example, examined health programs in faith-based organizations and their effectiveness and concluded that these settings can improve health outcomes. However, they also stress the need for innovative means of evaluating these types of programs.

Sternberg and colleagues (2006) review the literature on faith-based cardiovascular health promotion and identify a number of rewards and challenges associated with health promotion in these types of settings.

Trinitapoli (2005), in turn, found that religious congregations in general offer services for elders at lower levels than previous studies have shown, and even fewer services related to health promotion. Levin, Chatters, and Taylor (2005), in turn, caution the field not to foster unrealistic expectations of faith and spirituality in health and health-enhancement behavior. Jang, Borenstein, Chiriboga, Phillips, and Mortimer (2006) caution using religiosity across all African-American older adults who attend church. Instead, they found that religiosity and adherence to traditional culture influenced life satisfaction (psychological well-being).

Aaron, Levine, and Burstin (2003) conclude based upon their research that church attendance is a critical correlate of positive health care practices among African Americans. Idler (2006), in a review of the literature on religion and religiosity, found this construct to be multidimensional and quite complex, with different dimensions resulting in different health outcomes. Koenig (2003), in turn, found a strong relationship between health and faith, particularly for high-risk groups. This relationship extends beyond health seeking to include eating habits, exercise, smoking, alcohol use, drug use, sexual practices, sleep patterns, and driving safety, to list a few. Each of these behaviors has considerable consequence for a healthier lifestyle and health outcomes.

Not surprising, houses of worship have shown increased prominence as health promotion settings (Anderson, 2004; Lauder, Mummery, &

Sharkey, 2006; Tagilareni & King, 2006; White, Drechsel, & Johnson, 2006; Wilcox et al., 2007). Yanek, Becker, Moy, Gittelsohn, and Koffman (2001) report on the success of a cardiovascular program focused on African-American women. One study of urban women of color (Latina and African American) attendance at health clinics versus church-based exercise programs found that women aged fifty to seventy years old were twice as likely as any other age group to participate. Houses of worship, particularly in the case of Latinas, offered a viable setting for programs. Bullock (2006), in turn, highlights the potential of African-American churches in helping parishioners with advance directives, a topic rarely discussed in the literature. Waters (2000, 2001), too, stresses the potential of this setting to aid African Americans with end-of-life directives.

In the mid-1990s, Castro and colleagues (1995) reported on the use of Protestant churches to launch a peer-led health promotion program titled "Compañeros en la Salud" (Partners in Health). Peer-led health promotion programs such as this offer great potential, like their African-American counterparts, to reach Latino older adults with significant health care needs and limited access to bilingual and bicultural health information. Exploration of various points of entry into older adult communities of color provides the field with an expanded horizon for reaching them where they congregate and feel most comfortable and safe. In addition, these settings also provide health promoters with an opportunity to widen their initiatives to reach the family members of these older adults. These relatives are in an excellent position to reinforce the central goals of health promotion efforts.

Houses of worship have also been found to be an excellent resource for recruiting volunteers for various types of health initiatives (O'Neill, 2006–07). Zedlewski and Schaner (2006) found a strong relationship between formal volunteering and attendance in houses of worship. Houses of worship in urban communities of color rely quite heavily upon volunteers from their congregation to help carry out many of the social service activities often found in these settings. Thus, they also provide a strong base to find volunteers for health promotion projects, too.

Nevertheless, Ammerman and colleagues (2003), in a rare article on African-American church leaders and how they view church-university collaboration, raise the potential challenge of high pastor expectations in establishing collaborations based on research. Nevertheless, these high expectations may also be present in health promotion programming collaboration, making these types of initiatives challenging for health promoters wishing to engage these institutions. Koenig (2003, p. 963) concludes that houses of worship should not be overlooked by the field: "Yes, the faith community has a lot to contribute to the health and health care of our patients. How to sensitively and appropriately take advantage of this resource in terms of health education, disease screening, and health promotion will no doubt be a major challenge for our health care system in the 21st century."

Beauty Parlors and Barbershops

The use of beauty parlors and barbershops represents a new frontier in health promotion and human services in general. These institutions are often very well located within their communities, increasing physical access for urban older adults. Further, these settings are nonstigmatizing and are often staffed by community residents themselves who share the same cultural backgrounds as the clientele. These establishments meet the criteria that Delgado (1999) established for optimum urban nontraditional settings: (1) high volume of traffic, (2) time to actively engage a consumer, and (3) an atmosphere that is conducive for providing services.

Delgado (1997b), in a series of studies of Latina-owned beauty parlors, found these settings to be conducive for providing a wide range of psychological and social services that fall under the rubric of health promotion. Delgado (1999) also reports on a case study of Diana's Hair Ego (Columbia, South Carolina) of how a beauty parlor catering to a predominantly African-American customer base provides extensive health promotion services related to HIV/AIDS in this community, through public education and outreach. The American Society on Aging (2006) recommends that beauticians provide five-minute motivational talks on the virtues of proper diet and exercise for customers to address diabetes and other health concerns.

Hess and colleagues (2007) conducted two randomized feasibility studies involving barbershops and African-American/black males. The authors concluded that barbershops can function as effective hypertension detention, referral, and follow-up centers. Delgado (2007), in a study involving Latino barber shops as potential community sites for provision of a wide range of health and social services, found these settings to be ideal for reaching Latino males, particularly those who are older adults. Barbershops, like their female counterparts, can engage in health promotion activities targeting older adult males.

Food Establishments

The importance of proper diet within urban communities of color is well borne out in the research and scholarly literature, as noted in chapter 4. D. Gonzalez (2005, p. A25) comments on the consequences of poor health habits in New York City:

The devastating results of poor diet, no exercise and lots of stress are increasingly scaring health advocates in poor communities across the city. Diabetes is now the city's fourth leading cause of death. In neighborhoods where homicide or AIDS were the leading killers among young men and women a decade ago, heart disease and obesity are claiming ever more lives.

The lack of easy access (geographical and financial) to fresh produce and fruit, for example, is a critical ingredient in any social ecological approach to reducing overweight and obesity in the country (Galvez et al., 2008). Consequently, it cannot be considered a major stretch for health promotion initiatives to target these settings. In addition, food establishments within urban communities of color fulfill a wide variety of functions that are deeply steeped in cultural norms, beliefs, and attitudes, making these establishments of critical importance in the life of older adults and their families.

Grocery stores and restaurants, for example, can be found in virtually any urban community, regardless of the socioeconomic status of this community (Delgado, 1996). Their presence and easy geographical access make these institutions critical actors in health promotion initiatives that stress the importance of proper diet. Information pertaining to proper diet, for example, can be disseminated through these institutions. When this information is made available in the language and cultural background of the consumers, it takes on greater significance.

The high rates of diabetes in communities of color such as Latino communities, as already noted in chapter 4, have led Latino-owned bakeries to start making healthier versions of traditional Latino foods. Mi Vida-My Life Bakery, Santa Ana, California, for example, provides healthier variations of traditional Mexican baked goods, such as jalapeño tortillas, spinach tortillas, sweet concha pastries, and flaxseed bread, that are sugar-free and have lower carbohydrates, fat, and sodium (Benavides, 2005). Examples such as this can be found in increasing numbers across the country and open up the door for health promotion efforts to become even more community-centered by entering key institutions in the lives of urban residents.

Community Gardening

The reader again may be surprised by the inclusion of community gardens as a setting for older adult-led health promotion:

1. Gardening is usually not associated with urban areas.
2. Gardening is usually thought of as a means of beautifying sections of communities that have been consumed by "urban blight."

3. If and when community gardening is undertaken, it invariably is associated with a younger population group.
4. Gardening provides both a place and space for community-centered activities and interventions.

Consequently, the emergence of community gardening as a health promotion project has only recently in the last decade started to receive the attention it deserves from the field.

Urban planning and public health both share a primary goal of improving human well-being (Corburn, 2007; Fusco, 2007; Helwig, 2006; Hooker, Cirilli, & Wicks, 2007; Kochtitzky et al., 2006; Richard, Laforest, Dufresne, & Sapinski, 2004). Tzoulas and colleagues (2007) advance the concept of a "health ecosystem" (freedom from distress and degradation, maintains its organization and autonomy over time and is resilient to stress) and the importance of a relationship between green space and self-reported health. Cunningham and Michael (2004), in turn, in a review of the literature on the impact of the built environment on physical activity and older adults, found that the environment-behavior interaction in neighborhoods and this age group is still in its infancy, and inconsistent findings have made conclusive statements arduous. Nevertheless, the relationship between urban environment and older adult health has tremendous potential for the field.

The community gardening or greening movement provides the fields of public health, education, and human services, including health promotion, with a wealth of avenues for utilizing this vehicle to achieve goals related to well-being (Vasquez et al., 2007; Wakefield, Yeudall, Taron, Reynolds, & Skinner, 2007). Gearin and Kahle (2006) examined adolescent and adult perceptions of urban green space in Los Angeles and found differences in perceptions based upon age. Youth showed interests for socializing and relaxing while adults thought of green spaces as fulfilling recreational needs. E. N. Austin, Johnston, Yvonne, and Morgan (2006) advocate for the use of community gardening in senior centers as a means of increasing exercise and as a setting for developing community-based collaborations to encourage healthy lifestyles among older adults.

Heynen, Perkins, and Roy (2006) have found that greenery, in this case trees, positively affects the environment and is more often found in urban areas than in more affluent sections of a city, which tend to have lower percentages of people of color. Sullivan, Kuo, and Depooter (2004), in turn, come to the conclusion that trees and grass may be one of the key components of a vital community by facilitating social contact among neighbors. Baum (2002) recognized the potential of "greening" as a vehicle for helping older adults in health promotion. Residents living in relatively barren buildings and communities report greater incidents of anger and violence

(Kuo & Sullivan, 2001). Heynen and Lindsey (2003) use the concept of "urban canopy cover" as an indicator of the extent of greenery within a community. High indicators of greenery represent assets for urban communities.

Kweon, Sullivan, and Wiley (1998) specifically examined the potential role of green common space as a vehicle for socially integrating inner-city older adults and found that communities with green common spaces increase older adult social ties and create a positive sense of community. Although the movement toward creating greater green space in the nation's cities can be traced back over thirty years, the value and benefits of green space, and more specifically community gardening, is only now being fully appreciated within the health field.

The health promotion settings addressed in this chapter represent but the tip of what can be considered a sizable iceberg from a health promotion perspective. Embracing an assets perspective toward older adults and their communities represents the first significant step for the field for identifying potential health promotion settings for older adults and other population groups. The field is only limited by its imagination, and this is quite exciting and bodes well for its future. Further, the nature of health and its importance in the lives of older adults facilitate the emergence of initiatives that are not only consumer-created and led but also offer endless possibilities for a multidisciplinary collaborations pursuit of health from a social and economic justice perspective.

Some of these settings may hold great appeal for health promotion staff and the organizations that employ them; yet others may cause great trepidation and represent incredible challenges for which graduate school does not adequately prepare health promoters. That is natural. No one organization and staff can consider themselves to be in a position to try and engage all community-based health promotion settings that are "informal" in nature. Nevertheless, these nontraditional urban settings are quite conventional from a community perspective. Namely, they are organic or natural to the basic social fabric of the community and the world of older adults.

SECTION 3:
HEALTH PROMOTION
RESEARCH AND ETHICS

8

~

Research and Evidence-Based Older Adult Health Promotion

"The health promotion best practices literature is imbued with hope for knowledge mobilization, enhanced practice, and improved population health . . . health promotion is key to reducing the significant burden of chronic disease. However, we have seen little evidence of change."

(K. L. Robinson, Driedger, Elliott, & Eyles, 2006, p. 467)

The quote by Robinson and colleagues (2006) opening up this chapter highlights one of the key areas that will prove a formidable challenge for the health promotion field: the ever-increasing diversity found among older adults living in the United States. Barry and colleagues (2001), note, although referring to alcohol-related services but still applicable to other health-related topics, the importance of best practices for the field of health promotion:

We have moved into the 21st century with mandates to provide "best practice," guideline-driven care and at the same time to manage care in a cost-effective manner. Helping older adults who are at-risk drinkers to reduce or discontinue their use of alcohol is an excellent opportunity to improve practice care (p. ix).

The emergence of a best practice mindset and older adults brings with it much-needed attention to this field and age-population group, but also carries with this attention many of the challenges associated with better understanding what "best practices" ultimately means in the field of practice.

There is little disputing that health promotion is a complex topic that is made even more complex or challenging when applied to older adults.

161

This complexity, however, must not take away from the field's willingness, and ability, to conduct older adult health promotion. As noted in chapter 2, the health (economic, social, and political) of the nation rests in the balance as baby boomers continue to rapidly join the ranks of older adults. Concerted efforts to increase the health of older adults bring many benefits, including potential reduction of health costs and a potential volunteer force that can make significant contributions to their communities and to the nation as a whole. Probably most importantly, however, there is a positive qualitative change in quality of life for older adults who have historically been marginalized and suffered health ills throughout a major portion of their life.

Curry and Jackson (2003) argue that in order for scientific knowledge to advance regarding health disparities and older adults of color, these groups must be specifically targeted and systematically included in health research. Much progress has yet to be achieved in this area, however. Further, new models for both recruitment and active consumer involvement in health research are much needed to both increase our understanding of health disparities and result in the creation of health promotion interventions to address these disparities in a culturally competent manner. How best to capture this diversity and draw important implications for shaping older adult-led health promotion is no small issue.

Research will play an important role in helping the field to achieve the goal of making health promotion culturally competent (L. B. Wilson & Rymph, 2006). Further, as the field continues to expand its reach into new arenas to address health issues, such as many of those mentioned in chapter 4, it will need research that both captures emerging health issues for an increasingly diverse older adult population and documents successful strategies, activities, and tactics that can help develop new models that can be tested in multiple arenas. Nevertheless, this will necessitate coalitions and collaborations between academics, practitioners, and most importantly, consumers. Jamner (2000), as a result, strongly advocates for the introduction of innovative methods of research and program evaluation in community-based health promotion in order to fully capture the significance of this work in the community.

SAMHSA's Older Americans Substance Abuse and Mental Health Center (Blow, Bartels, Brockmann, & Van Citters, 2006) and the John A. Hartford Foundation (2005) note that evidence-based health promotion programs have played influential roles in shaping programming for older adults, and this bodes well for the field and the nation as a whole. Evidence-based health promotion has found its way into numerous areas such as smoking cessation (Abdullah & Simon, 2006), gambling (Desai et al., 2004), and alcohol and substance abuse (Barry et al., 2001). The list of subject areas will only increase in the foreseeable future, too, as the field of health promotion continues to expand its reach into previously over-looked health issues and problems among older adults.

The health promotion field has evolved over the past twenty-five years, and the importance of evidence-based practice has also evolved in parallel fashion to what has been experienced in other fields (Bunde-Birouste, 2002; Chwalisz, 2003; C. C. Collins & Benedict, 2006; J. Green, 2000; Koelen, Vaandrager, & Colomer, 2001; McNeill, 2006; Pynoos et al., 2006; Tagliareni & King, 2006). J. Green and Tones (1999), however, note that there has been a heavy influence of a biomedical agenda on evidence-based health promotion, and there is, as a result, a need for "judicial principle" (assembly of sufficient accumulated evidence) for assessing what constitutes evidence.

Evaluation of health promotion programs for older adults is very much guided by evidence-based principles and practices (Bryant, Alpeter, & Whitelaw, 2006). Bunde-Birouste (2002), for example, observes that the field of health promotion research and evaluation has made significant strides since its inception. However, it has not been able to maximize its potential because of an inability to influence key decision makers in the health arena. This argument can also be applied to the field as a whole and is certainly not restricted to one age group, such as older adults.

Valente (2002), in addressing health promotion evaluation, notes that four important factors need to enter into any research or evaluation effort: (1) an existing evidence base is utilized, (2) resources for the evaluation are available, (3) highly detailed characteristics of the health problem being addressed have been identified, and (4) characteristics of the target population are well developed. Valente's outline of the four key factors may seem straightforward to the uninitiated. However, each of these factors is fraught with complexities and challenges for the field of health promotion. When these factors are combined, the challenges facing academics and practitioners alike are formidable and not for the faint of heart. Yet, the most important step in addressing these complexities and challenges is recognizing them as such.

REWARDS AND CHALLENGES OF
HEALTH PROMOTION RESEARCH

Syme (2000) has recognized the charge often presented to the field of health promotion to be more innovative and rigorous in research design. However, this will require the field to improve on the current definitions of key concepts, in addition to improving measurement and assessment methods. One of the major barriers to this goal, however, is the manner in which "disease" is defined and classified, meaning the tremendous influence of a clinical model of disease. Rawson (2002), in turn, notes that health promotion is not a field that enjoys clarity and agreed-upon objectives, making technical application of scientific theory arduous to accomplish and creating a significant theory-practice gap: "For health promotion theory to be regarded as progressive it must be shown to accomplish all that rival approaches claim to plus it must uncover new possibilities for improving health or at least our understanding of what constitutes health. . . . This will be the most difficult aspect to establish but it would also generate the most powerful indicator for continued confidence in health promotion." In essence, extraordinary claims necessitate extraordinary results and documentation for the field, and older adults are not exempt from this challenge.

The rewards, challenges, and complexities associated with any form of evidence-based practice can also be found in the field of health promotion, including those focused on older adults, and particularly in cases where there is active engagement of program and community stakeholders (Bryant, Altpeter, & Whitclaw, 2006; Connell, 1999; Kahan & Goodstadt, 2001; Saskatchewan Health, 2003). However, N. Jackson and Waters (2005) comment on these challenges:

> Systematic reviews of public health interventions are fraught with challenges. Complexity is inherent; this may be due to multi-component interventions, diverse study populations, multiple outcomes measured, mixed study designs utilized and the effect of context on intervention design, implementation and effectiveness. . . . This necessitates expanding the traditional evaluation of evidence to incorporate the assessment of theory, integrity of interventions, context and sustainability of the interventions and outcomes (p. 368).

Thus, not surprisingly, the movement toward evidence-based practice in public health/health promotion has not escaped dilemmas, challenges, and debates (Ansari, 2005; Bunde-Birouste, 2002; J. Green, 2000; J. Green & Tones, 1999).

Allison and Rootman (1996), well over a decade ago, raised these challenges and debates pertaining to scientific rigor and health promotion research. More specifically according to Tilford (2000), debates have centered on two aspects: (1) what are the kinds of evidence utilized to determine effectiveness, and (2) what are the appropriate methodologies for developing such evidence? The content of these debates very often involves the role and degree of decision making that the consumer will have in dictating what information is important and what actions should transpire once answers are identified. The variety of health promotion goals also complicates the process of research and evaluation. J. Green and Tones (1999, p. 135) go on to comment: "Health promotion concerned with social and environmental change will clearly have different goals and different outcome indicators from those focused on individual behaviour change and or empowerment." Thorogood and Coombes (2004) note that the field has made significant progress over the past decade to address a variety of challenges, including the acceptance of a multifaceted approach toward evaluation of practice that stresses both quantitative and qualitative methods.

Tilford (2000) notes that the evolution of health promotion out of health education has been accompanied by a "time lag" in changing the proportion of evaluation interventions specifically focused on social determinants of health, rather than individual determinants usually associated with health education evaluation. Further challenges result from mistrust on the part of older adults of color regarding research of any kind, and more specifically, that focus on health (Moreno-John et al., 2004). Past negative experiences will shape current and future expectations.

Merzel and D'Afflitti (2003) undertook an extensive review of the literature on the evidence of community-based health promotion and concluded that the field faces significant challenges:

> The evidence from health promotion programs employing a community-based framework suggests that achieving behavioral and health change across an entire community is a challenging goal that many programs have failed to attain. . . . Methodological limitations, particularly issues related to low statistical power, impair the ability to detect significant differences, given the smaller-than-expected effect sizes typically obtained. These methodological challenges compound the difficulty of observing significant community-level changes in health behaviors when similar trends also are occurring in society at large (p. 571).

Kuller (2003), although acknowledging the challenges identified by Merzel and D'Afflitti (2003) and others, still stresses the need for the field to be able to achieve and document reduction of incidence or mortality of disease, or significant changes in risk factors, to be seriously considered as a viable intervention. McLeroy, Norton, Kegler, Burdine, and Sumaya (2003), in turn, argue that the field must adopt a widely accepted definition and typology of what is meant by the term *community-based* if it hopes to advance theory and knowledge on promoting health. The quest for consensus remains even though there are many in the field who would argue that it is and will remain elusive for the foreseeable future.

Finally, Nutbeam and Harris (1999, p. 64) put forth a perspective that is often overlooked in heated discussions about how best to support health promotion evidence-based practice: "Even the most causal observer of healthy public policy can see that there is often a poor relationship between what is known about factors that cause or could prevent illness and disability and the policies in place about these issues." "Evidence" as a critical factor in shaping health promotion is insufficient to move the field forward. The sociopolitical considerations wield tremendous influence on the extent to which evidence is considered sufficiently important to influence health promotion policy. As noted in chapter 5, health and illness are not apolitical constructs in our society.

CRITIQUE OF EVIDENCE-BASED
PRACTICE AND BIOMEDICAL RESEARCH

The upsurge in interest concerning evidence-based practice has not occurred without considerable debate or tensions over its evolution (Kahan & Goodstadt, 2001; Thorogood, 2002). Differences of opinion concerning how best evidence has been conceptualized and carried out can be seen in most, if not all, fields that have embraced this perspective. Critiques have generally fallen into various categories, with age-specific evidence being one of the most prominent. Bulatao and Anderson (2004), for example, recommend that health promotion research help inform interventions to more effectively reach the less-educated and low-income older adult of color. Delgado (2007), in turn, raises concerns about how best-evidence research has sought to homogenize Latino groups with very different sociocultural backgrounds and generalize findings to an entire group.

As with its youth-centered health promotion counterpart, differing ages within age groupings may respond differently to an intervention (Vasquez et al., 2007). Thus, the more specific the research concerning older adults, the more beneficial the results, and this necessitates that every effort be made to be group specific whenever possible to maximize health promotion initiatives. Consequently, when examining evidence-based practice, and the research that has effectively guided this social intervention, and marginalized communities, questions must be raised about the value of research findings based on one population group being generalized to other groups, such as older adults of color.

Koelen and colleagues (2001), in an extensive review of dilemmas and challenges related to biomedical-focused health promotion research, conclude that there are many limitations of using such designs in community-based health promotion because of the participatory philosophy inherent in most health promotion models. Biomedical-influenced health promotion research is based upon assumptions (clearly defined variables, measurable outcomes, and use of control groups) that effectively neglect meaningful community involvement in decision making. Further, the complexities associated with a socioecological perspective on health, as already addressed earlier in this book, necessitate the use of other methods or combinations of methods not normally used in biomedical-type research and evaluation. Consequently, knowledge gained on best practices using a biomedical paradigm is counter to what most progressive academics and practitioners say is needed to capture health promotion efforts that are consumer-driven or influenced.

However, this is not to say that counter arguments cannot be found in the field of health promotion. Sterman (2006), for example, argues that even though complexities hinder the field's ability to better understand interventions and unintended "side effects," this should not dissuade professionals from using systems theory and simulation modeling to broaden our options to generate and learn from evidence. Rosen and colleagues (2006), in turn, offer a strong defense of the virtues of utilizing randomized controlled trials in health promotion research. Although they acknowledge the widespread criticism of randomized trials, they contend that the limitations often associated with this research approach can be surmounted with "minor design" medications.

On a final note, Raphael (2000, p. 361) reminds the field that "evidence" is grounded within ideology, values, and principles and needs to be examined within this context: "Ideology, values and principles strongly influence what is accepted as valid evidence. Ideology is the world view or frame of reference that one uses to interpret a phenomenon." Thus, it is imperative that these elements be brought to the foreground in ascertaining what constitutes evidence and for whom. An embrace of evidence-based practice brings with it an implicit, if not explicit, acknowledgment that context must and needs to be made clear for evidence to be gathered and generalized for the field.

SELF/LOCAL KNOWLEDGE

Older adult-led health promotion is predicated on the value that older adults possess special knowledge of their situation or circumstance, which prepares them to better address health care needs. Unlike critiques involving youth self and local knowledge, older adults have had considerable years of experience that have provided them with a context upon which to judge and decide (Delgado, 2006). The concept of self/local knowledge brings older adults into direct conflict both with the prevailing wisdom of professionals and with who has the right to call themselves "experts" on older adults.

The devaluing of self or local knowledge by professionals can occur in a multitude of ways. However, it is probably most frequently done under the guise of the subject matter being addressed. The reader may be familiar with the argument that is often raised about how complex health is as a subject and the need for extensive formal education to better understand it. In essence, health care is best left to the "experts," or the "professionals." This argument, unfortunately, can be found in most learned gatherings. Nevertheless, that perspective, or belief system, creates a significant barrier between provider and consumer. Fischer (2003) notes:

> Many experiences from both social movements and institutionalized deliberative practices show citizens to be much more able to deal with complicated social and technical questions than the conventional wisdom generally assumes. . . . No case, for example, better illustrates such capabilities of citizens than the gay movement's struggle against the spread of AIDS (p. 148).

Older adult local and self-knowledge can be tapped in a variety of ways. For example, the use of a research advisory group composed of intended respondents has been used to assist in both the conceptualization of research methodology and questions, and the interpretation of findings among an urban-based group of Latino older adults (Delgado, 1997a). According to Delgado (1997a), the respondents were able to play a critical role in helping researchers better understand findings that were counterintuitive and thereby totally unexpected.

The construct of self/local knowledge is one that is particularly relevant when discussing older adult-led health promotion. Local or self-knowledge can be defined as "popular, or folk knowledge that can be contrasted to informal or specialized knowledge that defines scientific, professional, and intellectual elites in both Western and non-Western societies" (Brush, 1996, p. 4). Delgado (2006, p. 112) defines it thus: "In an age where expertise has become such a critical factor in determining social interventions, it is not surprising that the emergence of local knowledge as a key source of expertise has created such debate."

The concept of self-knowledge can be found in the professional literature in a variety of forms. In the case of older adults, not surprisingly, "wisdom" has emerged to capture this perspective. Edmondson (2005) notes that although the concept of wisdom and aging has been neglected in the twentieth century, its origins can be traced back to the Hebrew and Greek civilizations. Staudinger, Kessler, and Dorner (2006) advance the construct of wisdom (highest level of insight) among older adults, which represents a different way of looking at local knowledge or self-knowledge. Levy and Pilver (2006), however, caution about using this construct without engaging in stereotypes about older adults.

Local knowledge in its various manifestations requires that practitioners and academics develop a willingness and mechanisms for systematically tapping the voices and wishes of older adults regarding what it is that they want to get from health promotion initiatives, for example. Examples of this approach can be found in professional literature. Cousins (2003), for example, developed research that sought to uncover the "authentic views" of older adults on how they perceived physical activity, and found that promoting lifestyle changes is arduous to achieve without positive past-mastery experience. Greater understanding of older adult "self-talk," positive as well as negative, must be actively sought and taken into account in health promotion programming. Dunn and Riley-Doucet (2007) advance the use of discussion groups among older adults as a means of better grasping how lifestyles impact the physical, psychological, social, and spiritual health of this age group.

Fischer (2003), in his book on community and the environment and the politics associated with the debate between local knowledge and expertise (educational), brings to the fore the importance of citizens being actively involved in shaping policies and the barriers that they must overcome to have their voices heard and validated. Sirianni and Friedland (2001), in turn, also raise the need for communities to be empowered to shape public policy and the importance of the movement for civic renewal. Fischer (2003) has concluded that there is a tremendous need for active participation of citizenry in shaping environmental policy:

> Towards this end . . . experts have already innovated numerous techniques for facilitating the citizen's role in inquiry processes. The more critical question is how to bring these practices together in the professions. One of the most important points in the discussion of participatory inquiry has been the recognition that this involves more a question of attitudes and practices than matters of scientific methodology. Here we confront a matter of power relations as much as an issue of knowledge production (p. 260).

Sutton and Kemp (2006) advocate for the use of multidisciplinary knowledge and active community participation, which results in what they call "collective knowledge" and collective capacity to take action. Use of visualization tools, for example, helped community participants to better assess and understand local pressing issues and envision "novel solutions" to these issues. Professional-community collaboration efforts are not without challenges related to use of language (technical versus common), conceptualization of etiology, priority setting, and time intensity. Nevertheless, this should not serve as a detriment to collaborative efforts because of the inherent potential these efforts bring to health promotion and older adults.

Thus, if the means are there, then it is only a question of the political will to do so. In older adult-led health promotion, local knowledge shaped by years, if not decades, of experience with environmental justice issues (working within toxic environments as well as possibly living in toxic environments) can shape the will and the means for initiatives targeting environmental health issues. Older adults are in key positions to fill in the blanks on local history and events that have long gone unnoticed by the general public outside of the community. Their view of these events provides researchers with valuable insights into how the community views environmental justice issues, and can serve as catalysts for bringing about significant community involvement in addressing these sources of ill health.

PROMISING APPROACHES

It is appropriate to start this section with a quote by McLeroy and colleagues (2003) that, although it refers to public health in general, has particular meaning for the promise of health promotion:

> Public health is more than a body of theory and intervention methods. We cannot separate how we do public health from why we do public health. Whether we talk about changing behavior, changing community structures, or building community capacity, these changes cannot be separated from our ideals about what constitutes a good community or a good society (p. 532).

The concept of good community and good society captures the mission and goals encapsulated by older adult-led health promotion and the countless other promising approaches that have emerged in the past few years concerning the field of health promotion.

For example, the health promotion field has started to make important progress in developing research and evaluation methods that serve to increase older adult responses and participation in these endeavors. These advances, not surprisingly, have systematically sought to tap older adult voices in a manner that is empowering and culturally competent, and in the process of so doing, have provided important data for health promotion initiatives. Fischer (2003) notes:

> Indeed, distance has become the source of strident disagreements over the definition of the client's social situations, as well as over who should have the responsibility for determining the issue. Such struggles invariably raise the question of social control, typically leading to acrimonious polemics about the professional's role in the delivery of services (p. 183).

The report issued by the National Expert Panel on Community Health Promotion cited earlier in chapter 5 (J. L. Collins et al., 2007) recommends an increased commitment to community participation in public health research as a means of generating innovative health promotion programs.

Control, in effect, equates into power and decision making. In the case of conventional provider-consumer relationships, power rests in the hands of the provider. In older adult-led health promotion, it rests in the hands of the consumer. Abma (2005) puts forth the concept of responsive evaluation with values involving all stakeholders, including consumers, as a means of health promotion being able to address ambiguous contexts, as an example of power resting with the consumer. The emergence of the concept of "story harvesting" represents one qualitative method that has been successful in researching older adult women as used in the case study of the Older Women's Network presented in chapter 10. Pinn, Hill, Whitecross, Lloyd, and Pearce (2006, p. 19) note: "Using storytelling as a health promotion tool can take diverse forms. . . . The act of being involved in storytelling often provides a positive, healing and transformative experience, as well as the possibility of social change." Thus, this qualitative method not only informs practice with older adult women, but it can also result in social change brought about by participants, effectively eliminating the disconnect between research and action.

Cook (2007) advocates for the use of ethnography in health promotion as a means of decreasing the distrust of researchers and increasing the relevance of the findings for action. Goldman and colleagues (2003), in turn, strongly advocate for the use of a life history interview method to help capture the nuances associated with cultural belief systems for use in constructing health promotion initiatives targeting communities of color. This method, in addition, has particular relevance in the case of older adults of color because of the role and importance of oral history within many of these communities. This approach, although labor intensive and costly, will generate important information that would normally not emerge in a more conventional approach to data gathering. Further, it actively seeks to empower the older adult respondent in the process of gathering important information that is often either overlooked or completely lost in most conventional forms of research.

T. A. Baker and Wang (2006), too, stress the potential role of ethnographic (photovoice) participatory research methods. They used this method (photographs and narratives based upon their experiences with pain) to explore how chronic pain is experienced and dealt with by older adults. The use of photography and narrative taps into strengths that older adults possess in helping to shape interpretations of local conditions and circumstances from a historical perspective. Photovoice as a research method has been extensively used with youth (Delgado, 2006; N. Wilson et al., 2007). However, it is a method that is not age or group bound.

Hurworth, Harvey, and Rutter (2002) advance a model of evaluation involving older adults that is very attractive for the field of health promotion, particularly when initiatives are designed to be older adult led. This is a model that has been advocated for in youth-led health promotion (Delgado, 2006; Delgado & Zhou, 2008). However, it is rare in the case of older adults. Older adults can and must play an active and meaningful role in helping to shape evaluations of interventions that target them as beneficiaries. The field of health promotion with older adults has much to learn and gain from its youth-focused counterparts. Hurworth and colleagues (2002, p. 1) build upon the work of other scholars that stresses self-determination and enlightenment as key components of evaluation and apply them to older adults: "As a result of these aims of self-determination and enlightenment, empowerment evaluation is usually either for programs that assist disenfranchised or marginalized groups or for programs developed around social justice issues."

These authors identified eight key benefits that older adults derived from an application of empowerment evaluation in New Zealand–based projects:

1. Although initially suspicious, older adults eventually became active and meaningfully engaged.
2. The process of participating in interviews and training turned out to be more meaningful and enjoyable than initially expected.
3. Participants learned new skill sets.
4. Confidence and equality resulted from older adults working closely with evaluators.
5. Older adults accepted that they had a valuable role to play and contributions to make to the evaluation process.
6. A new strength of purpose resulted from teamwork.
7. Participants experienced new confidence in their abilities to undertake research and evaluation.
8. Participants played an instrumental role in lobbying local stakeholders regarding issues that were salient to them.

The case study presented in chapter 10 mirrors many of these and shows additional gains made by the women participants of the Older Women's Network.

The goal of using research and evaluation in empowerment approaches has been supported by the "democratization of science" movement. This movement has resulted in social activists across the entire life span influencing policies and funding of a range of public health issues related to environmental health such as asthma and breast cancer (P. Brown, 2007). "Lay" or consumer-professional partnerships have helped to expand the knowledge base on health and the environment, and also have resulted in health promotion initiatives that have been highly innovative.

The challenges related to undertaking research involving older adults of color are well understood in the field. Lack of trust in researchers is often the primary reason cited by experts, and this necessitates that trust building be integral throughout all phases of any research or evaluation endeavor (Lloyd et al., 2006). Development of trust is complex and reflects years of suspicion and negative experiences with having outside researchers enter their homes and draw conclusions that are detrimental to their community (Gamble, 1997). Once findings are uncovered, rarely does this information return back to the community in a manner that is affirming and of practice use.

Evaluation of older adult-led health promotion initiatives requires the development and use of culturally appropriate designs and methods to measure health-promoting behaviors, particularly in the case of groups that bring unique historical and cultural perspectives to definitions of health (Armer & Radina, 2002). Making comparisons across racial and ethnic groups utilizing "global" measures of health is not recommended, as noted throughout all portions of this book (Menac, Shooshtari, & Lambert, 2007).

Schensul, Disch, Vazquez, Radda, and Jepsen (2006) report on an innovative health promotion project that focused on urban older adults of color and their involvement in flu vaccination, with implications for research and program evaluation. Participants expressed a general willingness (90 percent) to inform other residents about flu vaccination opportunities. Further, 92 percent also indicated a willingness to participate in a flu surveillance project if requested to do so. The importance of flu vaccination has already been addressed earlier in this book (chapter 4), and this project attempts to overcome some of the barriers associated with such programs in urban areas with high numbers of older adults who are low income and of color. The peer influence of older adults informing other older adults addresses the potential they can play in health promotion education.

Last, Weitzman and Levkoff (2000), although specifically referring to a health dementia research study with elders of color, echo a theme found in most of the literature related to research of marginalized communities such as those of color, and that is the merit of combining qualitative and quantitative methods as a means of overcoming theoretical and recruitment problems. The complexities of the circumstances these groups find themselves in cannot possibly be understood and appreciated through exclusive use of one methodological approach. Multifaceted methods help increase the likelihood of the development of a comprehensive and in-depth understanding of health issues and the solutions that have the highest likelihood of achieving success.

On a less intensive level, there are interesting and innovative approaches that have started to find their way into the professional literature. The use of telephone and the mail system to track and reach urban population groups that are highly mobile have been found successful and offer potential for health promotion activities (Duffy, Goldberg, & Buch-wald, 2006; Napoles-Springer, Santoyo, & Stewart, 2005). These methods are relatively inexpensive and address very specific health promotion goals. Nevertheless, there are circumstances where older adults are home-less or do not have access to telephones, making these methods of limited use, particularly when taking into account literacy levels of older adults with limited formal educational backgrounds. The embrace of flexibility as a theme in health promotion programming allows the use of these and other unorthodox methods for the right circumstances. The same prin-ciple can also be applied to health promotion settings.

Older adult-focused health promotion, and particularly a model that stresses consumer-led leadership, places tremendous importance on listening to consumer voices and then systematically developing inter-ventions that build upon their cultural values, hopes, and expectations, and actively, and it meaningfully involves them throughout the entire process. The journey of gathering data is always fraught with challenges in any form of research. However, when discussing marginalized older adults, these challenges only increase in significance. Mistrust of outsid-ers, particularly those based in universities and representing dissimilar sociodemographic backgrounds to those being researched, have been well recognized in this chapter and countless other books related to re-search and communities of color.

These challenges or barriers, fortunately, can be surmounted through the embrace of participatory models that help provide venues for the voices of older adults to be heard and acted upon. Further, participatory models are not restricted to having older adults shape questions, meth-ods, and findings; they also can involve older adults playing the role of researcher in the process. This role has not received the attention that it warrants, but it does receive this attention in older adult-led health pro-motion.

9

~~

Ethical Dilemmas and Health Promotion with Older Adults

"'Health for all,' the universal vision that has guided health promotion efforts for the past two decades . . . envisages the attainment of a health level that permits all people to lead socially and economically productive lives. Yet we continue to live in a world with enormous health disparities."

(Marks & Shive, 2007, p. 28).

Social interventions are predicated upon decisions and alternatives that influence people; they necessitate value judgments to be exercised on what is perceived to be the "proper ethical" course of action that individuals and society must undertake. There is certainly a moral or philosophical basis to this form of decision making. In the case of health promotion, this judgment relates to what constitutes health and what are the "best" avenues to take to maintain it and rectify ill health when present (Naidoo & Wills, 2000). This perspective raises the importance of ethics and ethical dilemmas involving health promotion in general, and particularly when discussing marginalized older adults (Cribb & Duncan, 2002). The question at the heart of any ethical stance should be, "is what the field is promoting the 'best' that can be provided?" If the answer is no, then a series of ethical challenges can be levied that will challenge the very foundation upon which health promotion stands.

As the field of health promotion has gained national and international prominence, there has been a corresponding call for the introduction and greater prominence of ethics and ethical decision making into the field. The emergence of the Internet as a major source of information on self-care, for example, represents one of the latest advances in the field. However, with it there is a corresponding concern about the quality of health information that is available and the ethical issues this raises for those practicing self-care (Castiel, 2003). The emergence of technology and new ways of looking at health bring with it questions about ethics and ethical conduct, and this questioning is to be expected and encouraged across all facets of health promotion, including to what extent the ultimate beneficiaries of health promotion are playing a decision-making role.

In 2007, there was what might be arguably the first international conference specifically devoted to ethics and health promotion. "Setting an Ethical Agenda for Health Promotion" brought together an interdisciplinary gathering of academics and practitioners to examine the major ethical issues confronting the field and setting an agenda for better preparing the field to tackle these issues (Ghent University, 2007). This conference probably marks the first of countless other conferences to follow regarding health promotion and ethics and the need for all sectors, including consumers, to be a part of these types of deliberations.

The call for the recognition of ethics to play a more prominent and integral role in health promotion has been the result of concerns from the field, academia, and consumers about how ethical conduct must be systematically addressed as part of any aspect of health promotion practice and research. Coughlin (2006b, p. 827) for example, raises the constructs of hope and hopefulness applied to the area of ethics and health, with important implications for older adults who may be dying: "Although instilling false hope should be avoided, considerations of hope and hopefulness should figure more prominently in ethics frameworks and other conceptual models of public health practice. Sustaining or fostering hope among people and communities is consistent with the virtuous conduct of public health." Hope, as a result, enters into health care in a variety of ways that have ethical implications for social interventions such as health promotion (Simpson, 2004).

A number of important perspectives have recently emerged regarding ethics and health promotion. Marks and Shive (2007) have raised concerns about the existence and persistence of health inequalities in societies that have the requisite resources to eliminate these inequalities. Lewis (2001), in turn, uplifts the importance of definitions of "health" and "disease" in helping in ethical deliberations. Resnick (2007) notes that most of the attention in bioethics and health promotion has focused on society's obligations to provide health care. However, greater attention needs to be placed on strategies for addressing other dimensions related to health such as lifestyles. Lifestyles wield a tremendous influence on health, raising the importance of a social-economic perspective on ethics and health promotion. There certainly are no aspects of health promotion that are exempt from ethical decision making. Pauline, Pauline, Johnson, and Gamble (2006), for example, address the role of ethics and ethical issues related to exercise and health promotion, a topic that is generally not associated with ethics. Thus, there is no form of health promotion that does not touch upon some aspect of ethics and decision making.

VALUES AND ETHICAL DECISION MAKING

There is general agreement that any discussion of ethics and health must first require a discussion on what values underpin ethical decision making. Values such as freedom (autonomy), doing good (beneficence), doing no harm (nonmalfeasance), fairness (social and economic justice), and being true/honest (fidelity), for example, will quickly find their way into any serious discussion of ethics and health promotion (Castiel, 2003; MacDonald, 1998; O'Neill, 2002). These values, however, do not exist in a social vacuum, and this why ethical decision making is arduous: some of these values may conflict with each other from an institutional or practitioner point of view. Further, none of these values is more important than the others. These values, in addition, need to be grounded with a cultural context, increasing the importance of relativity depending upon the ethnic or racial group adhering to these values. Not surprisingly, these values do not share universal meaning and acceptance, and as a result, will engender great discussion and debate.

Minkler (2000), in addressing key values that wield tremendous influence in this nation, raises the challenges that they present to health promotion in its quest to embrace an expanded vision for the field:

> The dominant American self-image stressing individualism, self-reliance, and progress, and the "ethical individualism" to which it predisposes us makes our starting point on the road to a broader approach to health promotion a difficult one indeed . . . the time is ripe for considering broadening the ways in which we think about and approach health promotion (p. 372).

Ethical decision making, in essence, cannot be separated from the basic values that guide this nation and society, and as a result, the field of health promotion. The recent emergence of a journal titled *Public Health Ethics* (Oxford University Press) represents an example of how ethics has been elevated in importance in the field.

Ethics and ethical decision making and older adults have received increased attention in the health field. End-of-life care, for example, has probably generated the greatest discussion and scholarly attention regarding older adults (Raybould & Adler, 2006). Values pertaining to autonomy and informed consent, for example, often figure prominently in health care at this stage of life. Nevertheless, values based on autonomy and self-determination, like other values, are culture bound and often reflect an ethnocentric perspective that stresses individualization and less family and community-centered considerations.

Raphael (2000, p. 365) summed up quite nicely the value and importance of health promotion that integrates ethical principles: "There can be no better argument for health promoters to justify their activities than to state that not only is health promotion an ethical and principled discipline, but it is because of its value-based approach that it is effective." Thus, the clearer and more explicit the field is about the values that underlie urban-based older adult-led health promotion practice, the easier it will be to articulate the findings of these efforts.

Cribb and Duncan (2002) make the case for the importance of the field to systematically engage in debates about ethics and health promotion. The process of debating raises the likelihood that ethical decision making will be elevated to the point where ethics is discussed on a routine basis and integrated into everyday practice rather than relegated to special trainings and when circumstances dictate that time is set aside to address an ethical dilemma. Callahan and Jennings (2002), however, touch upon many of the challenges facing the field, including the importance of teaching ethics to professionals. The field of public health cannot take a perspective that is precise, particularly when it embraces a participatory approach toward research and program decision making, as noted throughout earlier portions of this book. However, many of the issues the field addresses do not lend themselves to this way of thinking about health and interventions.

ETHICS IN AN URBAN CONTEXT

It is impossible to examine health promotion and ethics without taking into consideration the context in which it occurs. A number of scholars in the fields of public health and health promotion have examined ethics, in this case bioethics, within an urban context. Blustein and Fleischman (2004) note that urban bioethics differs from traditional bioethics in two key ways:

> (1) examine[s] value concerns in a multicultural context, including issues related to equity and disparity, and public health concerns that may highlight conflict between individual rights and the public good, and (2) broaden[s] its primary focus on individual self-determination and respect for autonomy to include examination of the interests of family, community, and society (p. 1199).

This grounding within an urban context effectively opens ethics and ethical decision making to take into account themes of diversity, density, and complexity, which are often associated with urban living, and brings into any dialogue the importance of a social justice grounding and how the field must not shy away from such a sociopolitical perspective.

Fleischman and Barondess (2004) observe that the increased mortality among the urban poor has less to do with violence and substance abuse and more to do with diseases such as asthma, cardiovascular disease, diabetes, and kidney disease. The causes of these diseases have a great deal to do with racism, classism, and the lack of quality health care. As a result, these causes cannot be ignored in any meaningful discussion of ethics and health promotion. Health promotion interventions that ignore these causes of illness, in effect, can and should be questioned on ethical grounds.

Galea and Vlahov (2005, p. 341) pose provocative questions concerning health within an urban context, with implications for ethical decision making: "What then is urban health, and why should we concern ourselves with urban health as a specific subject of inquiry?" The responses to these two questions will undoubtedly vary from health promoter to health promoter and setting to setting. Nevertheless, regardless of the response, there is no denying that urban context profoundly shapes the health of city residents, and no more so than when discussing the most undervalued residents such as low-wealth/low-income older adults of color. Urban areas bring with them density, diversity, and complexity of living, and these three dimensions must be taken into account in any discussion of health promotion and ethics (Vlahov et al., 2007). Urban areas differ dramatically from rural areas of the country, and these differences get manifested in a multitude of ways. This geographical context, however, is further expressed when the population groups also differ dramatically based upon race and ethnicity.

The broad expanse of health promotion has necessitated that ethics and ethical decision making be taken out of a narrow focus on individuals and applied to more ecological environments. The influence of coalitions in urban-focused health promotion, for example, is a result of the shift that the field has experienced that has emphasized an ecological perspective on community and population groups. Wilken and Walker (2003), as a result, propose a ten-step decision making model that helps the field of health promotion in ethical decision making, in response to this need to view ethics beyond a focus on individuals. Adams and White (2005), however, raise a series of ethical concerns when a populations approach puts the health of easily identifiable individuals at risk.

The diversity found within urban areas in the United States must naturally weigh heavily on how ethics and ethical decision making gets conceptualized and carried out on a daily basis in health promotion programs targeting undervalued groups. Krumeich, Weijts, Reddy, and Meijer-Weitz (2001) stress the risk of ethnocentrism in undermining health promotion efforts targeting society's nondominant groups. The biases that emerge from an ethnocentric approach toward how health is defined and interventions conceptualized accordingly raise ethical issues for the field. Cultural bias is undeniable in any form of social intervention, and health promotion is certainly no exception. An ethical perspective, however, must enter into any dialogue about what is best for a population group that may not share a dominant worldview.

HEALTH PROMOTION ETHICS AND OLDER ADULTS

Health promotion's reach into specific population subgroups such as those who are youth, urban, low income/low wealth, and older adults, for example, has resulted in a realization that these and other population groups pose universal, as well as unique, ethical challenges for the field. Health promotion with older adults, for example, presents the field with a unique set of challenges or ethical dilemmas that can fall into many different categories or groupings. However, cultural bias against older adults from nondominant backgrounds such as those found in urban areas of the country that are low wealth/low income severely limits the effectiveness of health promotion (Bennett & Flaherty-Robb, 2003). The disconnect it causes regarding trust and communication, for example, often represents but the tip of the iceberg, so to speak, in barriers to effective health promotion.

There is a consensus that health promotion practice is complex and necessitates balancing scientific knowledge and participatory policy making, creating ethical dilemmas and a need for systematic ethical decision making (Weed & McKeown, 2003). Some of these ethical dilemmas are inherent in any type of health promotion effort, as already noted. However, some are very unique to the population group being addressed, as is in the case of low-wealth/low-income urban older adults of color. These older adults have significant barriers to overcome in achieving a healthy state of being. Consequently, extraordinary and innovative efforts must be carried out. Nevertheless, in the process of doing so, they both encounter and create ethical dilemmas for the field of health promotion that cannot be ignored.

Bennett and Flaherty-Robb (2003) conceptualize four issues affecting the health of older adults with implications for ethics and health promotion: (1) lack of resources, (2) scarcity of providers, (3) financial barriers, and (4) cultural barriers and biases. Each of these areas in isolation and in combination with each other is very applicable to urban-based, low-income/low-resource older adults. Ethics and ethical decision making, in turn, can also be viewed from each of these perspectives, providing the field a framework from which to better address ethical dilemmas and older adults. The four issues identified above share the need for the field to address discrimination as a central part of any intervention regarding marginalized older adults.

Coughlin (2006a), in an extensive review of the literature on ethical issues in epidemiologic research and public health practice such as health promotion, argues for the importance of the field paying greater attention to ethical issues in order to facilitate planning, implementation, and development of programs and research. Coughlin (2006a) goes on to differentiate between public health and medical ethics because the former has, among other differences, a broad emphasis that involves ethical and social issues such as those found in most forms of health promotion.

A focus on groups rather than individuals brings with it a perspective on ethics that generally stresses utilitarian decision making, such as the importance of aggregate or collective benefits to communities. Utilitarian theories that actively seek to incorporate principles of social and economic justice, as in the case of older adult-led health promotion, represent a natural way of viewing ethics and ethical decision making and cast this form of health promotion within a social backdrop that takes into consideration all of the forces that impinge on older adult health, including those that fall into a social justice viewpoint. Schroeder (2007), however, argues for a broader context beyond social justice as an ethical framework for health promotion and public health because reliance on this perspective is too narrow in focus and casts a multitude of factors that simply are not related to social justice into this category, thereby simplifying a very complex topic.

Hendricks, Hendricks, Webb, Davis, and Spencer-Morgan (2005) advance the notion that the field of health care has an ethical mandate to foster self-efficacy as part of its mission, although it brings with it a host of challenges. Older adult-led health promotion, too, seeks to foster self-efficacy, or empowerment, as a central goal. Hendricks and colleagues (2005) note:

> The continuous ethical challenge for health care providers, health promotion advocates and researchers is to remain mindful of the complexity of the opportunity to empower others, the privilege to improve the quality of life for others and the responsibility to remain true to the ethical principles at all times. Consideration of self-efficacy as an ethical mandate remains a vital element within health promotion practice and research (p. 1).

Consequently, practitioners who subscribe to this viewpoint have ethical obligations that can well be met through consumer-led health promotion efforts.

Lifestyle preferences bring an added and controversial perspective to health promotion and ethics, and unlike the issues raised with youth, older adults can engage in a wide variety of legal activities such as smoking, drinking, and gambling, for example. These activities, however, as already addressed in chapter 4, bring to the fore the role of responsibility and preferences to the field, and ethical challenges as a result. These and other activities can, and often do, have profound health consequences for older adults.

The field of health promotion has steadily made progress in introducing the subject of ethics as an integral part of the field. The subject of ethics, as a result, is no longer marginalized to the fringes of the field, although critics would argue that much more work in this area needs to transpire, particularly when addressing marginalized or undervalued groups in society. Bringing ethics and ethical decision making into a prominent part of any health promotion discussion is bound to cause tension and reduce the speed of any conceptualization and implementation of a project. However, this deliberation also helps to ensure that older adults of color are not relegated to second- or third-class status when discussing their rights and the benefits of participating in an intervention such as health promotion.

As this field continues to grow in importance and as health promotion ventures into generally unchartered waters involving new arenas, population groups, strategies, techniques, and settings, ethics will also evolve in helping the field navigate through turbulent waters. Ethics and ethical decision making specifically focused on older adults who are marginalized in this society will uplift universal ethical dilemmas associated with social interventions and undervalued groups. However, unique sets of ethical dilemmas will also appear regarding older adults.

The ethical dilemmas that were raised in this chapter, and the challenges that they pose for health promotion, can best be considered a starting point that will eventually evolve into the need for an entire book on the subject matter. Probably nothing less than a book can be considered satisfactory on a topic of such importance for the field of health promotion. Further, ethics and ethical decision making do not belong to any one group or arena, necessitating that all facets of the field of health promotion come together to develop and enforce ethical conduct by practitioners and academics alike.

SECTION 4:
REFLECTIONS FROM
THE FIELD

"Towns and cities should consider organizing large-scale, volunteer-based efforts that reach out to various sectors of their community in an inclusive way to identify and respond to the community's most pressing problems. The success of such efforts—involving individuals of all ages—is likely to depend on a leadership cadre of volunteers who are prepared to make it their principal activity. Once initiatives are designed with broad input, leaders can offer other volunteers a continuum of opportunities for involvement, ranging from episodic to regular and from causal to intensive."

(Center for Health Communication Harvard School of
Public Health, 2006, pp. 3-4)

10

⟍⟋

Case Study

"We must embark on a major marketing effort communicating that the aging of America is a great opportunity for individuals and society, a massive call to action that replaces the long-standing message that older adults are superfluous . . . with one that conveys to these individuals that they are not only needed but also have an essential contribution to make."

(Freedman, 1999, p. 233)

Freedman's quote sounds a call to action that effectively changes paradigms for how society views older adults and, in effect, how it needs to view the aging process. Such a call is nothing short of revolutionary in nature; make no mistake about it. There is little dispute that there often exists a formidable divide, or barrier, between the world of theory and academics and the world of practice. This lacuna has played a significant role in keeping fields from achieving their maximum potential since these two worlds must come together in order for practice to advance. The fields of gerontology and health promotion are certainly no exception. The emergence of the concept of "translation" has captured the importance of research findings being translated into practice in a timely and practitioner-friendly manner (Best et al., 2003; Oldenburg, Sallis, French, & Owen, 1999).

As noted throughout earlier portions of this book, concerns have been raised about how health promotion theory and research have been too slow in achieving this worthwhile goal. Case studies, however, have often served as field-based examples that lend themselves to translating theory and research findings into practice in a timely and effective manner. Some readers may even go so far as to start reading a case study in a book before reading all of the material leading up to this practice illustration. In these instances, the reader misses important foundation material leading up to the case study because of fears that the theory and research findings, particularly statistics, simply do not have relevance to their particular circumstance or situation. Most importantly, it also reflects a critical disconnect between academia and the practice world that effectively limits the field of health promotion from making significant inroads into marginalized urban communities and integrating cultural beliefs and attitudes that have historically been alien to this society and the field.

CASE STUDIES AND PRACTICE

Case studies have historically enjoyed a special place in the field of practice and continue to do so now. Case presentations, for example, are often utilized in the field as a mechanism for teaching and provision of consultation to organizational staff, and as a means of increasing the relevance of time spent on staff development. From an academic perspective, case studies have not enjoyed this appeal because of the interplay of a variety of key factors, particularly related to the generality of the findings. This limitation notwithstanding, case studies offer both academics and practitioners a domain where these two separate worlds can meet.

Case studies, however, have enjoyed some degree of acceptance in academic circles because of the "user-friendly" nature of the content being addressed. In essence, case studies facilitate translation of research into practice. This accomplishment takes on added significance in fields where social interventions are considered important. Case studies, as a result, are a mechanism or tool that can effectively weave together theory, research findings, and practical knowledge in a manner that is much more easily consumed by practitioners, although their value can also apply to consumers. Further, they serve as excellent teaching tools in the classroom. Thus, the reader can certainly appreciate why a case study has a prominent place in this book.

CASE SELECTION RATIONALE

There are tremendous amounts of considerations in the selection of a case study. The case must be significant for illustrating a particular concept or set of concepts; the availability of written documentation often facilitates the writing of a case study because it reduces the amount of time that goes into "recreating" history; the willingness of the participants to engage in dialogue is often a hindrance, particularly in cases where there is suspicion about academics; costs can be prohibitive; and finally, even though a case is particularly exciting for an author, that does not mean that this excitement is automatically translated into excitement for the reader. In essence, selection of case studies is both an art and a science, and like any subject that encompasses both of these spheres, there is considerable "wiggle room" in the selection process.

As a general rule, I always include a series of case studies in the books that I write. Such a goal is quite rewarding because it requires me to venture out into the field in an attempt to make a book as relevant and reader-friendly as possible. However, I often struggle with finding the "perfect" formula for presenting case studies in a book. A principal struggle often centers on the number of cases selected for inclusion. Presenting multiple cases provides the reader with an opportunity to examine theory and practice from a variety of perspectives and settings. This enriches a book because it allows an author to highlight the breadth of a field. However, in doing so, depth is often sacrificed for breadth. Presenting one case study, in turn, allows an author to provide a wealth of information and allows a reader a chance to fully appreciate the multitude and magnitude of factors or circumstances, as well as the context of the case being presented. However, the breadth of a field is sacrificed in the process.

I have elected to go the route of selecting one case study to highlight in this book. The significance of the case that was ultimately selected will not be lost on the reader. The wealth of written information and evaluation data combined with the cooperation of the participating parties, even though they were almost halfway around the world in Australia, made the decision easy to make. As the reader will see, the Older Women's Network (OWN) provides richness in detail, and their perspective on health and wellness within a social and economic justice context brings attention to the plight of women as they enter old age.

Although every effort was made to find a case study of an urban-based older adult-led health promotion program in the United States, I was not successful in doing so. In fact, I had to leave the country and hemisphere to find an older adult-led health promotion program that provided the necessary richness in history, structure, and documentation for inclusion in this book. Mind you, this is not to say that there are no such type programs in the United States that were equally worthy of this attention, because there no doubt certainly are. Unfortunately, I could not find one. Nevertheless, the selection of OWN for this book, I am confident that the reader will agree, is quite special.

OLDER WOMEN'S NETWORK,
NEW SOUTH WALES, AUSTRALIA

History/Rationale for Establishment

The birth of OWN can be traced back over twenty years (1986) as an indigenous effort to develop a support group for and by older women. OWN was originally established in New South Wales, Australia. New South Wales is Australia's most populated state with almost seven million inhabitants. Sydney is the capital, with almost 63 percent of the state's population calling it home. The impetus for the development of this organization was the self-help movement and its potential to enrich the lives of older adult women and their communities. Like other self-help movements, it actively sought to empower participants and challenged stereotypes of older adults and their capabilities to effect change in their lives and their surrounding world. Self-help groups such as OWN undergo an evolution in how the group or organization views itself and its relationship to the external world. However, it never loses sight of the impetus for its establishment.

Mission

The Older Women's Network mission statement provides the reader with a vision of the organization's values and purpose (Older Women's Network, 2006b):

> The Older Women's Network (OWN) works to achieve a caring society in which older and midlife women have the opportunity to live in security and with dignity; to participate in the choices affecting their lives; to give mutual support and share creative interests and activities; and to realize their potential. OWN is a VOICE for older and midlife women in our changing, diverse [Australian] society; one which changes discrimination on the basis of age, gender, sexual orientation, race, ethnic origin, religion or disability. OWN is an EDUCATIONAL ORGANIZATION which embraces a feminist perspective in order to empower women to overcome injustices and inequities in the home, in the workplace and in the large society.

This mission statement provides a socioecological perspective that addresses the key barriers that older women often face in seeking wellness, as well as the multiple levels of discrimination that older women who are not white or heterosexual face in having their needs met in society in a manner that is reaffirming of their identity. The importance of empowerment in achieving a healthy state of being, as addressed throughout early portions of this book, is critical in shaping how participants view the organization and, in this case, the role of gender and how older adult women are undervalued and stereotyped by society. This sociopolitical context cannot and should not be ignored by older women if they wish to seek to maintain an identity that is affirming and brings hope of a state of well-being that takes into account their unique circumstances in society. A feminist and social justice perspective effectively grounds all facets of how health is defined and successfully addressed in a society that consistently marginalizes women, particularly those who are older adults.

OWN Definition of Health

The definition of health that follows effectively serves to ground the OWN mission within a broad and multifaceted understanding of health, or wellness, which is social, cultural, economic, and political in nature, and highlights this from a gender, or feminist, perspective. OWN's definition of what constitutes health captures how health is defined in this book quite eloquently, as noted in chapter 5 (Pinn et al., 2006):

> The OWN Model of Wellness is a concept of health promotion designed by older women for older women to increase and develop the wellness of older women. Wellness emphasizes lifestyle and well-being rather than illness. The aim of wellness activities is to give back to older women a sense that they can live with fullness and richness in their life. Wellness is about having a balance between the physical, emotional, social, intellectual, and spiritual aspects of life. It implies a positive attitude, strength of mind, and captures the essence of women participating, playing, acting, working, contributing to and enjoying life (p. 5).

The multifaceted perspective on defining wellness, or health, reinforces the central tenets of OWN and reinforces many of the key themes raised throughout this book on the need for older adult health promotion to ground interventions based upon how older adults view and define the meaning of health. It is no mistake that OWN's embrace of an ecological view of health grounds this definition within a social and economic context, and how ecology influences health and provision of quality care. The introduction of spirituality into this definition reflects a growing trend in the field of gerontology and stresses the need for a definition of health that goes far beyond the traditional boundaries associated with a medical definition of health.

Guiding Principles

OWN's eleven guiding principles cover a wide range of areas and serve to both embrace and express a core set of values and beliefs that guide the organization's activities and empower participants. These guiding principles bear a tremendous resemblance to the older adult-led principles identified in chapter 6. The guiding principles that follow are well grounded within the existing literature on social and economic justice and ecologically focused health promotion (Older Women's Network, 2006b):

1. **Recognition of Older Women**: Older women have the right to be valued and recognized for their contribution to the political, social, and cultural areas of life. Older women should have the opportunity to participate in all aspects of decision making that could affect their well-being.
2. **Our Environment**: The Older Women's Network understands that the environment is not just a physical issue. The environment is an all-encompassing concept that influences, and is influenced by, economic, social, cultural, and psychological factors such as housing, transport, health, social justice, education, and the mass media.
3. **Health**: Health is more than just the absence of disease. Health also includes a personal sense of well-being. Socioeconomic, emotional, social, cultural, and physical factors influence health and well-being. The Older Women's Network believes that priority must be given to the maintenance of health and the prevention of illness.
4. **Violence and Abuse**: The Older Women's Network believes that freedom from violence and abuse is a basic human right. Violence and abuse includes: neglect; physical assault; psychological, emotional, and verbal abuse; sexual assault and abuse; financial and economic exploitation; and social abuse.
5. **Home, Community, and Residential Care**: The rights of older women to define their own needs and to choose appropriate care and support services are essential to their dignity and well-being.
6. **Discrimination**: The Older Women's Network is committed to the elimination of all forms of discrimination but particularly discrimination based on age, gender, and race.
7. **Transport**: Affordable and accessible public and private transport is essential for older women to maintain their independence and to avoid social isolation.
8. **Education**: Older women learn and develop a wide range of skills throughout their lives. It is vital that older women have access to learning activities that enable them to keep pace with change to enhance self-fulfillment and to continue their contribution to community life.
9. **Income Security**: The Older Women's Network recognizes that a majority of women throughout their lives are disadvantaged in making provision for their financial security in later life. In addition, government policies can impact adversely on the incomes of older women. To maintain quality of life, health, and well-being, it is vital that older women have a base of retirement income that is adequate to their needs.

10. **Housing**: Older women have a right to safe, secure, appropriate, and affordable accommodation.
11. **Carers**: The Older Women's Network recognizes the importance of ongoing support services that address a variety of needs an[d] issues relevant to voluntary carers' lifestyles and particular needs. These include adequate financial assistance, access to quality respite care, information, education and training, emotional support, and community involvement.

The eleven principles outlined above provide the reader with a comprehensive understanding of how the health of one older adult group, in this case one that is female, can encompass social, economic, political, and psychological dimensions. In addition, these principles reflect a keen understanding of how social and economic justice forces have shaped how older adult women have seen their state of health compromised by social and economic environmental factors. Each of these principles addresses a particular aspect of health, but when combined, they provide a powerful view of how health must be defined and addressed by society when specifically focusing on a marginalized group such as older women.

OWN Management

OWN's self-help philosophy wields a tremendous amount of influence on how the program gets managed on a day-to-day basis. In 2007, twenty groups or chapters, each with a volunteer coordinator serving an elected term of office, comprised OWN NSW (New South Wales). OWN NSW, in turn, is managed by a team of thirteen members, six of whom are from outside of the metropolitan area. Day-to-day coordination is done by a coordinator group that is composed of three members from the management team. Participatory democracy principles guide the selection of managers and their decision-making process and actively seek to broaden leadership opportunities.

Membership

Membership characteristics, not surprisingly, vary considerably according to the location of OWN's Wellness group or center. The most diverse center had a membership of 57 percent with cultural and linguistic backgrounds other than white. The average age of members also differed, with one center having an average age of 78 for its members. OWN activities, as a result, are available in a variety of languages such as English, Arabic, Greek, and Vietnamese, for example. One center, for example, found that over half (52 percent) of its members spoke a language other than English at home.

Programming and Activities

The importance of programming being flexible, consumer driven, and sensitive to socioecological forces has been stressed throughout this book, particularly in chapters 5 and 6. OWN's Wellness programming or services to older adult women are characterized by flexibility in level and type of participation. Wellness groups are formed around a variety of consumer-driven activities, most notably physical movement; film discussion groups; health information sharing; group discussion of a variety of subjects, speakers, creative opportunities, and structured social relations. Activities such as attendance at rotating different local restaurants; cruises; quilting; bingo; African drumming; music concerts; anniversary group celebrations; celebrations of International Woman's Day and Mother's Day; community tours of radio stations, town halls, libraries, and botanical gardens; support groups for cancer survivors and those with depression or anxiety; swimming; aqua-aerobics; tai chi; *feldenkrais*; drumming; dancing; and singing typify physical activities that cater to different participant interests and abilities. Media coverage is important as a means of both increasing the visibility of OWN to attract new members as well as increasing public awareness and support of organizational activities.

Participants also can take part in lunch and coffee exchanges. Social opportunities, in addition, transpire during the planning of events and activities outside of the group such as movies, theater, and worship services. Participants can engage in any of the above planned activities or as many as they feel comfortable doing or as their schedules permit. It is not unusual, for example, to have new members start with one activity and, as they increase their comfort level, expand to include other activities and possibly positions of leadership.

OWN also publishes a monthly newsletter titled *OWN Matters*, which is available in paper form as well as online through OWN's web page. This newsletter provides OWN with an opportunity to share with members and those outside of the organization information regarding projects, activities, and schedules. It also provides members with a venue to share narratives, poems, and stories. One section titled "OWN Advocacy" shares reports and information on social activism undertaken by OWN on behalf of women and health. An annual conference is held that members from all OWN groups to attend.

Civic engagement opportunities, as addressed in chapter 3, can also take on a variety of manifestations, with OWN members engaging in local politics, speaking at conferences, assuming membership on boards and on the management team, reflecting well on members progressively increasing the nature and extent of their participation. Social activism represents a natural extension of civic participation and empowerment and the embrace of a socioecological view of health (Pinn et al., 2006, p. 59): "For many their activism began with their Wellness group. They were concerned with more than their own wellness and were advocates for the wellness movement and for securing the sustainability of groups by obtaining funding. They were advocating the need for more government support, to maintain what exists and to expand Wellness groups and activities." This activism, however, also extended beyond the confines of Wellness groups and encompassed community health–related issues and concerns.

There has been a concerted effort to expand the traditional base of membership. Although OWN is composed of older adult women, the organization has established a Younger Older Women's Group for members as young as fifty years of age in an attempt to provide support for women in this age grouping. The Aboriginal Support Circle (ASC) represents a major initiative on the part of OWN to address the needs of women of color. This diversity initiative/programming was established in 1994.

A socioecological perspective toward health and health promotion requires a deep understanding of the origins and causes of health disparities. ASC's origins are based upon an understanding of the deleterious consequences of social and economic injustices perpetuated by the "invasion of Australia by white people [and how] the indigenous people of Australia have been subjected to seizure of their land, attempted genocide, loss of diversity, persecution and gross discrimination"(OWN, 2006a, p. 2.) The ostracism of Aboriginals, like the experiences of people of color in the United States, has resulted in health and social inequalities. Greater awareness of Aboriginal history, customs, and cultures represents an initial and important step toward achieving reconciliation and wellness.

The aims of the ASC are as follows (OWN, 2006a):

> The overall aim of the OWN Aboriginal Support Circle is to study Aboriginal history, customs and culture with a view to extending this knowledge to family and friends so that a better appreciation of Australian indigenous people will be gained. Our specific aim is to use this knowledge and understanding to cultivate a better relationship and friendship with older Aboriginal women so that we can work together to add value to the lives of older women in Australia (p. 1–2).

ASC activities are multifaceted:

1. use of Aboriginal women as guest speakers
2. participation in reconciliation events
3. visits to Aboriginal communities
4. organized trips to important Aboriginal sites

5. attendance at cultural Aboriginal events
6. participation in events sponsored by the Council for Reconciliation
7. use of music, poetry, and humor to convey serious messages
8. monitoring of discriminatory practices by media and in policy documents
9. undertaking research to enable members to understand broader issues
10. supporting Aboriginal organizations through attendance at meetings and rallies and lobbying on behalf of Aboriginal people
11. supporting Aboriginal organizations and events with financial contributions

These activities address the importance of increasing public awareness of the plight of Aboriginal women, but they also encourage advocacy on behalf of and social action involving Aboriginal people.

Funding

The challenge of finding funding sources that bring with them minimal political and administrative "strings," particularly documentation of services demands, is a perennial challenge in Australia as well as other countries throughout the world. Self-help efforts invariably function with low budgets and, as a result, rely heavily upon volunteers and in-kind contributions, and OWN's funding base represents this position quite well. OWN funding comes from a variety of sources such as membership fees (these fees represent a very small percentage of the annual operating budget), the NSW Department of Aging and Disability Department and Wellness Project, and the NSW Department of Health. The City of Sydney provides space for OWN in a variety of sites. Bequests are also solicited. A shift toward "conventional" sources of funding, in turn, necessitates greater emphasis on evaluation documentation to be provided that highlights the success of a program, as noted in the following section.

Evaluation

In the spirit of older adult empowerment, the Older Women's Network relied heavily upon a participatory approach toward evaluation of its programs, and this entailed having organizational members play a central role in all facets of the evaluation process. The evaluation was characterized as being with, rather than on or of, program participants, different from conventional evaluations that do not actively involve the beneficiaries of the services in decision-making roles.

1. **Main Focus of Evaluation and Coordinating Team**: The evaluation of OWN focused on three critical programmatic themes (Pinn et al., 2006, p. 21): "the wellness groups and their activities, what wellness means to the participants, and personal stories of developing wellness." These three areas of focus provided both process and outcome data that not only served to gather data on program performance but also empowered participants in the process.

   The coordinating evaluation team consisted of fourteen members (twelve women and two men), with older women program participants consisting of half (seven members) of the team. The remaining team members consisted of five health professionals and two university researchers. Evaluation fulfilled a variety of key functions in addition to providing data on the success of the Wellness groups. Evaluation also served as an empowering mechanism for OWN women to take greater control over their own destinies within and outside of their participation in the program.

2. **Training and Support of Participants**: A participatory evaluation undertaking usually involves a large number of program participants to fulfill a wide range of roles, and the OWN evaluation was no exception. This necessitated that careful planning and requisite resources be devoted to preparing participants to play active and meaningful roles in the evaluation effort. Evaluation staff consisted of twenty program participants and health professionals.

   The training covered a two-day period and addressed the following (Pinn et al., 2006, p. 21): "Provide an overview of story harvesting as an approach to evaluation; allow for collective design of the guiding questions to be used in harvesting stories; provide an opportunity to learn about, and practice, semi-structured interviewing and the facilitation of group storytelling; and allow people to understand the application of ethics to this form of evaluation." Harvesting of stories was undertaken through one of four approaches to maximize flexibility in older women telling their stories in a manner that best suited their individual talents:
   i. a recorded conversational approach based on a one-to-one format utilizing semi-structured interviews
   ii. recorded group discussions
   iii. use of creative methods such as poetry, painting, songwriting, and collages
   iv. use of e-mail and other written forms of expression for those who preferred to share their stories while alone

This flexibility in approaches touched upon an important theme related to older adult-led health promotion by recognizing the myriad of ways that older adults communicate their perspective on health based upon their cultural backgrounds and how they, in turn, conceptualize health. Interestingly, only two participants submitted visual expressions and three submitted poems. Nevertheless, the option of utilizing unconventional approaches to eliciting responses is important in all facets of older adult-led health promotion, including evaluation. A willingness to explore innovative approaches is exciting, and this is contagious and opens up new venues for data gathering that is highly sensitive to contextual setting.

Training also emphasized ethical conduct and decision making, including the use of a consent form, protection of data, confidentiality and anonymity of the participant stories used to illustrate key themes, and review of the evaluation process by an institutional review board (Sydney Health Ethics Committee). Ethical considerations, as a result, were an integral part of the evaluation effort and stressed participation and decision making on the part of participants.

3. **Data Analysis**: Analysis of data, too, followed a collaborative and participatory process by actively engaging older adult participants playing a role in all facets of data coding and analysis over a two-month period. The analysis uncovered seven key themes. Each theme that follows, in turn, was manifested along social, emotional, physical, mental, spiritual, skill, and participatory dimensions, taking into account an emphasis on empowerment principles (Pinn et al., 2006, pp. 77–83):
    i. Wellness groups provide a gateway for older women's journeys into wellness.
    ii. Wellness activities enable women to challenge stereotypes of older women.
    iii. Wellness groups' culture of acceptance and self-direction is central to wellness.
    iv. Support for lifelong learning is a vital aspect of wellness activities.
    v. Social action, advocacy, and active citizenship develop through wellness activities.
    vi. Epiphanies lead to transformative understandings about wellness.
    vii. Expressions of wellness are complex and often paradoxical.

The findings of OWN's evaluation effort reflect well on the organization's attractiveness to participants' operative reality as it pertains to health in context. Further, the findings stressed the importance of lifelong learning and the role it can play in helping participants better understand and appreciate their abilities to learn, grow, and share in a collective and interdependent manner. Last, social activism has the potential to involve participants along a continuum of activities that facilitate participation according to the goals and comfort levels of members. Self-determination is a powerful mechanism for engaging members and helping them determine their individual and group goals.

Future Plans

The future potential of OWN goes far beyond the original geographical boundaries of Australia and the English-speaking world. The principles upon which OWN is founded are universal with equal applicability to other parts of the world. Thus, its potential for expansion across countries and hemispheres is limitless, particularly when it can adapt to local circumstances.

It is fitting to end this section of the OWN case study with a quote by Renate, an OWN evaluation team member talking about the promise of collaborative research, and a central theme of this book (Pinn et al., 2006):

> I always wondered whether true collaborative research was somewhat of a pipe dream. One could get close to it, but there had to be a little hint of hierarchy. Now I know it can happen and I am so lucky to be part of it. The miracle has happened on both sides—the fact that the bureaucrats, the academics and the consumers could be so completely and excitedly on the same wavelength seems like the most amazing part of the experience (p. 30).

Case studies fulfill such important functions in bringing together theory and practice. The case of OWN, I believe, does a wonderful job of illustrating the potential of the field of older adult-led health promotion to make significant contributions both nationally and internationally. Further, it opens the door for other innovations such as older adult-led research and community organizing, for example, which allow the field to continue its reach into population subpockets that have suffered as a result of a history of neglect, with health disparities being but one dimension of the consequences.

OWN has evolved over the years to encompass a more comprehensive perspective on older adult women's health and health promotion, and this is clearly the mark of a successful program. Further, the program has not been satisfied to rest on its accomplishments and has instead pushed the boundaries of what constitutes an older adult health program, in the process making important contributions to other consumer-led health program initiatives. Most importantly, OWN has shown the world (policy makers, academics/researchers, and consumers) what is possible when health is defined in a holistic fashion and interventions are conceptualized as broad and multifaceted. Older adult-led health promotion involving collaboration between consumers, practitioners, and academics is not only possible but also highly recommended. An embrace of participatory democracy and empowerment principles effectively serves as a bridge or Rosetta stone for facilitating communication between different worlds, so to speak.

Finally, it is fitting to conclude this chapter and case study with a quote from one of the OWN members (Pauline), since the organization is all about and for its members (Pinn et al., 2006):

> Even just the discussions we've had I've quite enjoyed. . . . I must admit now, while it isn't a physical activity, as far as I can see the communication skills are just as much part of your physical [wellness]. They're more your spiritual and emotional well-being—to hear what other people have to say, to hear what their lives have been like as well. I think I value too the openness of most of the women that I've met, the general acceptance (p. 36).

Older adult-led health promotion is about connectedness, empowerment, and having a sense of purpose, and not just physical health or the absence of disease and illness. Pauline's observations of what OWN has meant to her brings this important point to the fore, and it is one that must not be forgotten by the field!

11

⁓

Future Rewards and Challenges for the Field

"Finally, the development of effective health promotion will require health professionals with new skills. These skills include an ability to analyze health problems at various levels of social organization, re-frame health problems to engage diverse constituencies in the health promotion process, advocate for policy change in the face of opposition by special interests, and evaluate the success of health promotion inter-ventions that seek changes in fundamental determinants."

(Freudenberg, 2007, p. 2)

As is customary in my books, the final chapter provides me with an opportunity to both reflect on key themes that emerged during the writing of the book and raise important challenges that remain un-addressed by the field and are, as a result, inherently tension producing. There are tremendous opportunities as well as challenges for the field of older adult-led health promotion. The rewards and challenges that follow represent the most important ones facing the field. Of course, they represent the views of just one individual and there are, no doubt, countless other perspectives on what are the most pressing rewards and challenges.

The Ottawa Charter for Health Promotion (1986) uplifts the value of a healthy citizenry to a society.

Health is created and lived by people within the settings of their everyday life; where they learn, work, play and love. Health is created by caring for oneself and others, by being able to take decisions and have control over

199

one's life circumstances, and by ensuring that the society one lives in creates conditions that allow the attainment of health by all its members (p. 3).

The rewards of health promotion for individuals, communities, and society, are self-evident. However, reading the following challenges may result in feelings of hopelessness or even anxiety. The challenges, however, must be viewed as opportunities for the field to make significant and lasting strides in the future.

The eleven points that follow, I believe, uplift for dialogue the major rewards and challenges facing the field of health promotion as it contemplates its future in the early part of the twenty-first century and how well it will embrace or reject older adult-led interventions. The following issues touch upon theoretical, social, economic, political, and methodological forces that all converge to challenge the field of health promotion to better address the needs of marginalized urban-based older adults, and to do so in a manner that is participatory and empowering in the process.

1. Who Owns Health Promotion?

Clearly, no profession should "own" this field. The complexity of the field has only increased this past decade, and there are no reasons to suspect that it will stop in complexity in the next decade. This multidisciplinary view of health promotion, when combined with a participatory set of values and principles, means that a partnership between professions (academics as well as practitioners) and community, in this case older adults, is not only necessary but critical in importance. The importance of health in the lives of individuals and their communities is such that a nation with a large proportion of its citizenship unhealthy is a nation in serious decline globally. Further, the richness resulting from the interchange of disciplines is simply not possible when one discipline dictates how health promotion is conceptualized, implemented, and evaluated.

Rather than having a discipline/professional ownership discussion or debate, it is recommended that we view this from a consumer perspective, having older adults, in our case, decide who is able and willing to collaborate with them on health promotion. Mind you, I am not naïve about the political and funding importance of a particular discipline "owning" health promotion. Prestige and resources are part of the important gains that result from such ownership. Lobbying for funds is often one of the critical functions of a profession. However, the community ultimately loses in the case of low-wealth/low-income urban older adults. Their needs and circumstances are great, and so are their assets. The type of health promotion advocated for in this book necessitates a team/coalition approach that places older adults front and center in decision making. What better goal is there than to decide who is allowed at the table to work with older adults and to have these older adults set the agenda? Consumer-led health promotion is just that—the ultimate beneficiaries decide who they want to collaborate with, how, and when.

2. Evidence-Based Practice, but Whose Evidence?

Health promotion, older adult-led or otherwise, will need to come to grips with the power of evidence in moving forward in the next decade. Evidence-based practice has achieved incredible momentum this past decade, and it would be foolhardy to ignore its importance in academic and funding circles. However, this does not mean that we naturally assume that "others" or "experts" are in the best position to decide what is "worthy" practice from a research or evaluation perspective. The process used to determine what measures are indicative of "best practice" is even more important than the actual outcomes because they ultimately decide what is, and is not, important to know.

How can older adults help move this discussion forward? I believe that they are the ultimate judges of what evidence is important in their lives, and we as providers and academics must follow suit and develop measures that help capture what older adults believe is important. The reader who adheres to a set of values and principles that reinforce the importance and authority associated with educational expertise legitimacy (university degrees) will surely disagree with this recommendation. Older adult-led health promotion stresses the importance of experiential expertise (living the experience or walking the walk) versus learning about the experience in a classroom. These are certainly two different worldviews that must be reconciled if we are to agree on what constitutes evidence in older adult-led health promotion! In many ways, this represents the process associated with a journey rather than a destination.

3. Diversity Brings with It Rewards and Challenges

The field of health promotion has embraced the importance of context, with culture being one key element, and this embrace has also opened up a complex set of challenges. The increasing diversity found among older adults (racial, ethnic, geographical, sexual identity and orientation, acculturation level, etc.), is exciting for the field because it opens the door for the introduction of innovation in how to conceptualize and deliver health promotion. At the very least, it certainly brings the need for variety and flexibility into health promotion activities. However, it also brings with it the potential for tension and strong differences of opinions concerning where and how health promotion targeting older adults can and should transpire. Mind you, this tension is not limited to older adults and can be found in other age groups, too.

These tensions and differences must be viewed as normalized and thus part of the process of designing and implementing older adult-led health promotion. Thus, older adults harbor attitudes that can be considered racist, classist, and homophobic, for example. Growth is an ongoing process and does not stop at any particular age, and lifelong learning is not limited to academic-related knowledge and can also apply to attitudes. Consequently, it would be foolhardy to think that older adults do not have strong biases that effectively limit their engagement of adults from disparate backgrounds. This acknowledgement becomes important and presents an opportunity for older adults to expand their vision of other individuals who are different from themselves.

4. Specificity Is the Name of the Game

Terms and concepts play such an important role in the field of health promotion. Terms such as "older adult," "people of color," "marginalized," "undervalued," "urban resident," and "minorities," are too general in nature to be effective categorizations of people for health promotion. All but the last term has been used throughout this book to facilitate delivery of content. In "real life," however, it is necessary to be much more specific about age, socioeconomic status, gender and sexual orientation, acculturation level, and religious affiliation and practices, to list but a few key factors in the planning and delivery of older adult-led health promotion.

This perspective on specificity leads to clarity concerning intent and outcomes of health promotion initiatives, but it will also do wonders for facilitating development of measures for assessing outcomes when evaluation occurs. Terms often enjoy different meanings within and between professions, even in different parts of the country, and this diversity of opinion can also be found among consumers. Consequently, older adult-led health promotion, like many of its counterparts involving other sociodemographic groups, must strive to arrive at a consensus whenever possible on the key concepts and terms that are integral to this movement. The process of arriving at a consensus and greater clarity can serve many important purposes beyond facilitating research and evaluation. This process will undoubtedly also uncover different assumptions, or biases, into which those practicing in the field probably had little insight. Further, the process is probably as important as the outcome and thereby should not be short-circuited for the purposes of expediency.

5. Aging as a Normative Process

Older adults, regardless of their social circumstances, must not be categorized as a "social problem" for the nation, and must also resist being relegated to having their "problems" solved through "medical" interventions in the process. C. D. Austin (2005, p. 307) sums up this challenge quite well in the following assessment. "My view is that the biggest challenge we face is the medicalization of aging, the continued transformation of growing older into a series of diagnostic categories, organ systems, diseases to be conquered, and drugs to be administered; the dominance of curing over caring." The "medicalization" of aging, incidentally, will put older adults of low income/low wealth at a distinct disadvantage when compared with their wealthier counterparts, further increasing health disparities because of limited access to quality health care.

Growing old is a privilege rather than a curse. If older adults internalized a view of themselves as being cursed, then it would be a monumental challenge to see themselves as possessing the necessary skills to bring positive change to the field of health promotion, or any other field. Older adults are their own best advocates and are in the best position to change attitudes. At the very least, they are instrumental members of teams and coalitions; preferably, they are key decision makers. Their worldly experiences should be tapped by succeeding generations and society as a whole. Unfortunately, we live in a society that systematically segregates its population based upon age. There are very few places in a community, other than houses of worship and possibly libraries, where multiple generations can attend together. This is in sharp contrast to many different cultures where older adults are integral parts of families and institutions. The debate about old age, as a result, must shift and embrace terms and symbols that are affirming and empowering.

6. Older Adults: Can't Live with Them and Can't Live without Them!

Society can ill-afford to cast aside a significant portion of its population (and an ever-increasing proportion at that) and not suffer severe economic, political, and social consequences. When a society actively marginalizes another age group, as in the case of youth, for example, it is destined not to last. In the case of older adults, unlike their youth counterparts, they have the right to vote in public elections and, in the case of a select subgroup, control a great deal of wealth. These two so-called considerations wield a considerable amount of influence in helping to shape how elected leaders view this constituency.

Thinking of older adults as a national resource or, dare say I, treasure, helps reshift society into thinking of this age group as a social capital to be nurtured and utilized effectively and efficiently. The emergence of a construct such as civic engagement provides both a conceptual under-pinning and "currency" for many of the nation's leading think tanks to promote ways that older adults can continue to be productive citizens in innovative ways, as noted in chapter 5. Participation on the part of older adults, however, must not be measured solely by the increased numbers of participants but also by the quality of the opportunities made available to them to lead and engage in active decision making. Participation by itself is an important criterion, but assessing the quality of that participa-tion has far-reaching implications.

7. Academics: Can't Live with Them and Can't Live without Them!

There is no disputing that academics have historically been viewed with great suspicion by marginalized urban communities, and for very good reason. We have reputations of entering these communities and gathering the information (data) that we and our funders believe to be important, and then leaving without any direct and immediate benefit to these com-munities. Further, to add insult to injury, we have relied upon deficit paradigms and written scholarly publications casting aspersions on many undervalued groups, particularly those of color. Consequently, raising the question, "Is there a role for academics in older adult-led health pro-motion?" is not without merits.

Although it may be difficult for some practitioners and consumers of health care to appreciate, academics can have an important role to play in older adult-led health promotion, as noted by Freudenberg (2007, p. 2): "By framing health as an economic, environmental, social justice, and moral issue, health professionals can enlist more stakeholders in the process. Academics can contribute to this goal by studying the process of health mobilization and identifying the characteristics of effective strategies."

Freudenberg's (2007) assessment of the academy and health promotion may appear foolhardy from a practitioner's perspective based upon their experiences with academics doing work in undervalued communities. However, health promotion addressing any age group necessitates a team approach, including having the consumer be a key member, and in the case of older adult led, a principal decision maker. Galea and Vlahov (2005) stress the importance of cross-disciplinary collaborations in any effort to address urban health. "Urban health promotion," for example, provides an opportunity to create a common language that facilitates collaboration that seeks to marshal complementary skills. Collaboration must be broadly defined to go beyond professionals and disciplines to also include consumers and communities.

Academics, it should be emphasized, often have the time, funding, and access to institutional resources that can be marshaled in service to a community. When discussing undervalued or disenfranchised communities in this society such as older adults of color with low wealth/income, all resources that can be tapped must be tapped, including those in academia. We in academia, in turn, must be able to join forces with practitioners and consumers without attitudes of superiority, which is so often the case, and even in professions that ostensibly seek to provide social assistance to those in greatest need.

8. Social Justice versus Economic Imperative

Older adults are often mentioned as potential detriments to society's economic well-being. The great debates pertaining to how the country's social security system will be bankrupted in the next twenty or so years are rarely countered by a social justice perspective concerning the rights and privileges of older adults. If society can systematically and structurally find avenues for incorporating older adults into its basic fabric, then this debate becomes superfluous, so to speak. The so-called "burden of support" is erased to one of shared responsibilities and mutual concerns. The future, after all, is not the exclusive domain of any one age group. If you are alive, then you are part of the future!

No sector of society should be relegated to its margins for any reason, least of all a developmental phase that most human beings secretly strive to achieve if they are lucky. Aging is a natural phenomenon that is not unique to our society and culture, and our society must reshift its thinking about older adults. Our society has much to learn from cultures that revere the older adult members of their community. Strictly viewing the value of a human being based upon their economic abilities to produce highly valued goods and services is a very narrow view. The social climate of a society that embraces all age groups will have tremendous implications for health well-being, not to mention social well-being. The case example presented in chapter 10 is illustrative of the importance of social and economic justice serving as a context and guide for better understanding health and illness.

Social and economic justice is premised on the importance of human rights being validated and protected. The oppression of any one group, such as older adults, for example, effectively means that any group is capable of being oppressed because of their social characteristics or values. Consequently, an open and affirming embrace of social and economic justice principles necessitates that older adult-led health promotion integrate social activism into the fabric of any intervention. Social activism, in turn, can take on a wide variety of formats depending upon local goals and circumstances. Embracing social activism, however, will have a direct consequence on the nature of organizational funding that is sought because of potential political backlash on the organization.

9. The Case for Urbanized Health Promotion

The importance of context in the form of geography and culture, for example, in shaping older adult health promotion is well established in the field, although there still is much more progress to be accomplished in this area. This approach, however, does have its critics who may favor not separating out older adults based upon a host of sociocultural factors for fears that doing so undermines their political influence and negates their commonality in the process. Nevertheless, urban older adults who are of color and low income/low wealth bring to the field a unique set of rewards and challenges that their rural, white, non-Latino counterparts do not.

The high concentration of older adults in cities provides the field of health promotion with an excellent opportunity to initiate programs that reach out to countless numbers of older adults who are clustered, or are segregated as the case may be, within communities. Further, the field is able to initiate programs that cut across different ethnic and racial groups that can serve as models for reaching other age groups. Urbanized health promotion will eventually evolve into its own specialty group, so to speak, that can be found in journals, conferences, workshops, and funding streams, just like it has in the broader field of public health and social work. This will probably occur in the next decade as the field continues to evolve into subspecializations that are geographically or population bound. Developmentally, this will bode well for the field because it will serve to attract scholars and practitioners with this particular context as their primary site for delivering health promotion. This does not mean that the field will become segmented or fragmented to the point where subspecialties go their own way. It does mean that annual conferences on health promotion, for example, will have universal as well as specialty tracks that address the general field as well as special interests.

10. Wellness Promotion

The emergence of a "wellness" or "successful aging" construct represents a shift in conventional thinking about health promotion from a deficit (disease and illness) to one of enhancement and opportunities (Albert, 2004; Jamner & Stokols, 2000). Although the concept of wellness has achieved broad if not universal appeal, its definition, like that of health promotion, is still ambiguous (Breslow, 2000, p. 41): "Wellness as a health goal is still a relatively crude concept. It has not yet become sufficiently explicit and standardized to permit clear delineation in a person or measurement in a population." Nevertheless, disease prevention and wellness promotion are considered the two critical aspects of a positive health strategy (Breslow, 2000).

This lack of consensus on what wellness means has facilitated the use of this concept in a multitude of ways. Wellness promotion, for example, is often associated with older adults (Brewer, 2004; C. A. Miller, 2003) and stresses activities and interventions that are nonstigmatizing for participants. Nevertheless, the concept of wellness seems to be very closely tied to higher socioeconomic groups, and its potential to reach undervalued older adults such as the ones discussed in this book remains to be fully realized in the field. In essence, is "wellness" a construct that explicitly or implicitly refers to the "worthy" older adults or can it also be applied to those older adults for whom a wellness construct is simply out of the question? Unfortunately, the axiom that wealth buys health is very much a part of the wellness movement as it is now conceptualized, although the reader may disagree with this assessment.

In the Older Women's Network's embrace of wellness represents a political discussion that emphasizes the need to better understand what this term means within a sociocultural context and gender. Wellness is a multifaceted construct that can and must be grounded within a social and economic justice set of values and also grounded within a social determinant of health perspective.

11. Older Adult-Led Health Promotion Is Great, but Who Is Going to Fund It?

The value of health promotion across the entire life span is pretty well established from a well-being perspective. The economic value in savings to employer and government (tax payer) is also is increasingly less debatable. Thus, if everyone is in general agreement that health promotion, and in the case of this book, that targeting older adults, is a win-win for older adults and society, then why is it so difficult to find a source of public funding that can sustain and even enhance this movement? There is no secret that the prevention field has historically found it difficult to find a steady source of funding. After all, it is so much easier to document the solving of problems rather than the preventing of problems, and this is certainly the case when examining marginalized communities such as low-income/low-wealth older adults of color concentrated in the nation's inner cities.

Health promotion's primary goal of saving the tax payers' dollars is misguided but still has value (Cohen & Hale, 2002):

> Economics provides the framework for considering how efficiently health promotion achieves its objectives and how health promotion resources can be used most cost-effectively. Economics also provides an analysis of health-promoting behaviour and of the incentives that exist to prevent ill health or to engage in activities that damage health (p. 178).

However, it would be foolish for the field to place cost saving as the primary goal because an increase in quality of life cannot be measured by dollars alone. Healthy older adults do not live in isolation from other age groups. The increase in well-being in one age group will undoubtedly have a ripple effect upon other groups (close friends, family, and community). Measuring the impact of a healthy state of being in older adults must not be narrowly conceptualized.

Funding, as evidenced by the Older Women's Network case, is a perennial challenge. The source of the funding becomes of greater importance than the actual amount of funding. Funding that severely restricts activities or necessitates extraordinary efforts at maintaining documentation (paperwork) can severely curtail the potential of the organization's seeking to redress the consequences of oppression. Development of a multifaceted funding base in which less than one-third of all funding comes from a highly restrictive funder, in turn, necessitates organizations' developing the capacity to undertake this type of funding. This is certainly not an easy challenge for any organization, least of all one that is self-help oriented.

There are numerous lessons that have been learned over the decades pertaining to older adults, health, and peer-led health promotion efforts. First and foremost, it is important to note that older adult-led health promotion should not be viewed as a panacea for all of the health needs confronting this age group. Chapman and Pancoast (1985), almost twenty-five years ago, raised the important conclusion, which is also applicable to the model put forth in this book, that older adults providing services cannot be a substitute for formal services. In essence, older adult services, in this case health promotion focused, must be conceptualized as part of an array of services, some conventional or traditional with professionals providing the leadership, and others more innovative with varying degrees of older adult leadership, including older adult-led.

No field worth its salt, so to speak, can be considered significant without its share of challenges and controversies. Insignificant topics do not warrant close scrutiny, and as a result, debates. Older adult-led health promotion is sufficiently challenging to warrant serious discussion of what this model means for the fields of health promotion and gerontology, as well as the nation. Thus, it is appropriate to end this book on the importance of debate in the field. Some readers may not like this. However, the field of older adult health promotion, and in this case, older adult-led, is too important to avoid possible tensions. The benefits of this attention will spill over into health promotion and other population groups. These groups, too, will benefit, and so will the nation!

Bibliography

Aaron, K. F., Levine, D., & Burstin, H. R. (2003). African American church participation and health care practices. *Journal of General Internal Medicine, 18*, 908–913.

Abdullah, A. S. M., & Simon, J. L. (2006). Health promotion in older adults: Evidence-based cessation programs for use in primary settings. *Geriatrics, 61*, 30–34.

Abma, T. A. (2005). Responsive evaluation in health promotion: Its value for ambiguous contexts. *Health Promotion International, 20*, 391–397.

Achenbaum, W. A. (2006). Civic ventures: Looking backward, planning forward. *Public Policy & Aging Report, 16*, 9–12.

———. (2006–07). A history of civic engagement of older people. *Generations, 30*, 18–23.

Acton, G. L., & Carter, P. A. (2006). Health promotion research: Addressing the needs of older adults and their caregivers. *Journal of Gerontological Nursing, 32*, 5–11.

Adams, J., & White, M. (2005). When the population approach to prevention puts the health of individuals at risk. *International Journal of Epidemiology, 34*, 40–43.

Aday, R. H. (2006). Aging prisoners. In B. Berkman & S. D'Ambruoso (Eds.), *Handbook of social work in health and aging* (pp. 231–241). New York: Oxford University Press.

Adler, G., & Rottunda, S. (2006). Older adults' perspectives on driving cessation. *Journal of Aging Studies, 20*, 227–235.

Adler, P. A., & Roberts, B. L. (2006). The use of Tai Chi to improve health in older adults. *Orthopedic Nursing, 25*, 122–126.

Adler, R. P., & Goggin, J. (2005). What do we mean by "civic engagement?" *Journal of Transformative Education, 3*, 236–253.

Adlong, W. (2006). Framing participatory inquiry in terms of "reflexivity." *Proceedings of APEN International Conference*, March 6–8, 2006, Beechworth, Victoria, Australia.

Administration on Aging. (2004). *Older women.* Washington, DC: U.S. Department of Health and Human Services.

AGS Foundation for Health in Aging. (2006). *Among frail older adults, increased age, loss of strength, and curtaining living situations are associated with the decision to stop driving.* New York: Author.

Albert, S. M. (2004). *Public health and aging: An introduction to maximizing function and well-being.* New York: Springer.

Alkema, G. F., & Alley, D. E. (2006). Gerontology's future: An integrative model for disciplinary advancement. *The Gerontologist, 46,* 574–582.

Allegrante, J. P. (2006). In search of a new ethic for health promotion. *Health Education & Behavior, 33,* 305–307.

Allen, A. (2001). Developing an innovative fall prevention strategy in a primary care setting. In A. Chiva & D. Stears (Eds.), *Promoting the health of older people* (pp. 99–111). Buckingham, England: Open University Press.

Allison, K. R., & Rootman, I. (1996). Scientific rigor and community participation in health promotion research: Are they compatible? *Health Promotion International, 11, 333–340.*

Almqvist, L., Hellnas, P., Stefansson, M., & Granlund, M. (2006). "I can play!": Young children's perceptions of health. *Pediatric Rehabilitation, 9,* 275–284.

Altman, D. G., & Sevick, M. A. (2002). Book review of D. R. Buchanan (2000). An ethic for health promotion: Rethinking the sources of human well-being. *Health Education Research, 17,* 134–138.

Altschuler, J., Katz, A. D., & Tynan, M. (2004). Developing and implementing an HIV/AIDS educational curriculum for older adults. *The Gerontologist, 44,* 121–126.

American Medical Association. (2003, March 19). Public health and aging: Trends in aging—United States and worldwide. *Journal of the American Medical Association, 289,* 1371–1373.

American Psychological Association. (2003). *Mental health care and older adults: Facts and policy recommendations.* Washington, DC: Author.

———. (2004). *Fostering resilience in response to terrorism: For psychologists working with older adults.* Washington, DC: Author.

American Society on Aging. (2001). *Literature review and selected biography: Barriers to older adult health education.* San Francisco: Author.

———. (2006). *Diabetes prevention and management.* San Francisco: Author.

———. (2007). *About ASA's Civic Engagement Program.* San Francisco: Author.

Ammerman, A., Corbie-Smith, G., St. George, D. M. M., Washington, C., Weathers, B., & Jackson-Christian, B. (2003). Research expectations among African American church leaders in the PRAISE! project: A randomized trial guided by community-based participatory research. *American Journal of Public Health, 93,* 1720–1727.

Anderson, C. M. (2004). The delivery of health care in faith-based organizations: Parish nurses as promoters of health. *Health Community, 16,* 117–128.

Andrews, C. (in press). An exploratory study of substance abuse among Latino older adults. *Journal of Gerontological Social Work.* (forthcoming)

Aneshensel, C. S., Wight, R. C., Miller-Martinez, D., Botticello, A. L., Karlamangla, A. S., & Seeman, T. E. (2007). Urban neighborhoods and depressive symptoms among older adults. *The Journals of Gerontology Series B: Psychological Sciences and Social Sciences, 62*, S52–S59.

Angel, J. L., & Angel. R. J. (2003). Hispanic diversity and health care coverage. *Public Policy & Aging Report, 13*, 8–12.

———. (2006). Minority group status and healthful aging: Social structure still matters. *American Journal of Public Health, 96*, 1152–1159.

Angel, J. L., & Whitfield, K. E. (Eds.). (2007). *The health of aging Hispanics: The Mexican-origin population.* New York: Springer.

Ansari, W. E. (2005). Collaborative research partnerships with disadvantaged communities: Challenges and potential solutions. *Public Health, 119*, 758–770.

Arcury, T. A., Bell, R. A., Vitolinas, M. Z., & Quandt, S. A. (2005). Rural older adults' beliefs and behavior to complementary and alternative medicine use. *Complementary Health Practice Review, 4*, 33–44.

Arcury, T. A., Grzywacz, J. G., Bell, R. A., Neilberg, R. H., Lang, W., & Quandt, S. A. (2007). Herbal remedy use as health self-management among older adults. *The Journals of Gerontology Series B: Psychological Sciences and Social Sciences, 62*, S142–S149.

Arean, P. A. (2003). Advances in psychotherapy for mental illness in late life. *American Journal of Geriatric Psychiatry, 11*, 4–6.

Arean, P. A., & Unutzer, J. (2003). Inequalities in depression management in low-income, minority, and old-old adults: A matter of access to preferred treatment. *Journal of the American Geriatric Society, 51*, 1808–1809.

Arif, A. A., Rohrer, J. E., & Delclos, G. L. (2005). A population-based study of asthma, quality of life, and occupation among elderly Hispanic and non-Hispanic whites: A cross-sectional investigation. *BMC Public Health, 5*, 97.

Armer, J. M., & Radina, M. E. (2002). Definition of health and health promoting behaviors among Midwestern Amish families. *Journal of Multicultural Nursing, 8*, 43–52.

Aspinalla, P. J. (2007). Language ability: A neglected dimension in the profiling of populations and health service users. *Health Education Journal, 66*, 90–106.

Associated Press. (2007, September 29). Aging inmates clogging nation's prisons. Retrieved September 29, 2007, from www.usatoday.com/news/nation/2007-09-29-aging-inmates_N.htm.

Austin, C. D. (2005). Not just another population. *Families in Society, 86*, 307–308.

Austin, C. D., DesCamp, E., Flux, D., McCleland, R., & Sleppert, J. (2005). Community development with older adults in their neighborhood: The Elder Friendly Community Program. *Families in Society, 86*, 401–410.

Austin, E. N., Johnston, E. N., Yvonne, A. M., & Morgan, L. L. (2006). Community gardening in a senior center: A therapeutic intervention to improve the health of older adults. *Therapeutic Recreation Journal, 40*, 348–351

Ayalon, L., & Arean, P. A. (2004). Knowledge of Alzheimer's disease in four ethnic groups of older adults. *International Journal of Geriatric Psychiatry, 19*, 51–57.

The baby boomers' tab. (2006, July 17). *Toronto Star*, p. A15.

Baker, D. L. (2001). Reducing falls among older adults residing in the community. In E. A. Swanson, T. Tripp-Reimer, & K. Buckwalter (Eds.), *Health promotion and disease prevention in the older adult: Interventions and recommendations* (pp. 119–126). New York: Springer.

Baker, D. W., Gazmararian, J. A., Sudano, J., & Patterson, M. (2000). The association between age and health literacy among elderly persons. *The Journals of Gerontology Series B: Psychological Sciences and Social Sciences, 55,* S368–S374.

Baker, D. W., Wolf, M. S., Feinglass, J., Thompson, J. A., Gazmararian, J. A., & Huang, J. (2007). Health literacy and morality among elderly persons. *Archives of Internal Medicine, 167,* 1503–1509.

Baker, R. (2005). *The hidden epidemic: Older individuals with HIV infection.* Retrieved October 8, 2007, from www.HIVandHepatitis.com

Baker, T. A., & Wang, C. C. (2006). Photovoice: Use of a participatory action research method to explore the chronic pain experience in older adults. *Qualitative Health Research, 16,* 1405–1413.

Bandura, A. (2004). Health promotion by social cognitive means. *Health Education & Behavior, 31,* 143–164.

Bandura, A., & Schunk, D. (1981). Cultivating competence, self-efficacy, and intrinsic interest through proximal self-motivation. *Journal of Personality and Social Psychology, 41,* 586–598.

Barry, K. L., Oslin, D. W., & Blow, F. C. (2001). *Alcohol problems in older adults: Prevention and management.* New York: Springer.

Bartles, S. (2003). Improving the system of care for older adults with mental illness in the United States: Findings and recommendations for the President's New Freedom Commission on Mental Health. *American Journal of Geriatric Psychiatry, 11,* 486–497.

Bassey, W. P. (2003). HIV/AIDS case profiles of African Americans—Guidelines for ethnic-specific health promotion, education, and risk reduction activities for African Americans. *Family Community Health, 26,* 289–306.

Bauer, M. J., Rottunda, S., & Adler, G. (2003). Older women and driving cessation. *Qualitative Social Work, 2,* 309–325.

Baum, P. (2002). Health and greening the city: Setting for health promotion. *Journal of Epidemiology and Community Health, 56,* 897–898.

Beattie, B. L., Whitelaw, N., Mettler, M., & Turner, D. (2003). A vision for older adults and health promotion. *American Journal of Health Promotion, 18,* 200–204.

Beck, J. C. (2000). Preventing disability in older Americans: The challenge of the 21st century. In M. S. Jamner & D. Stokols (Eds.), *Promoting human wellness: New frontiers for research, practice, and policy* (pp. 424–462). Berkeley: University of California Press.

Becker, G., Gates, R. J., & Newsom, E. (2004). Self-care among chronically ill African Americans: Culture, health disparities, and health insurance status. *American Journal of Public Health, 94,* 2066–2073.

Bedard, M., Stones, M., Guyatt, G. H., & Hirdes, J. P. (2001). Traffic-related fatalities among older drivers and passengers: Past and future trends. *The Gerontologist, 41,* 751–756.

Bell, R. A., Suerken, C. K., Grzywacz, J. G., Lang, W., Quandt, S. A., & Arcury, T. A. (2006). CAM use among older adults age 65 or older with hypertension in the United States: General use and disease treatment. *The Journal of Alternative and Complementary Medicine, 12,* 903–909.

Belyea, M. J., Pierce, M. B., & Lamwi-Keefe, C. J. (2003). Nutrition, older adulthood. In T. P. Gullotta & M. Bloom (Eds.), *Encyclopedia of primary prevention and health promotion* (pp. 736–741). New York: Springer.

Belza, B., Walwick, J., Schwartz, S., Shiu-Thornton, S., & Naylor, M. (2004). Older adult perspective on physical activity and exercise: Multiple cultures. *Prevention of Chronic Diseases, 1*, A09.

Benavides, D. (2005, August 3). Living la vida buena: Mi Vida-My Life bakery targets Latino shoppers with healthier versions of traditional Mexican goods. *The Orange County Register.* Retrieved November 6, 2007, from www.ocregister .com/ocr/sections/business/business/article_620000.php.

Benisovich, S. V., & King, A. C. (2003). Meaning and knowledge of health among older adult immigrants from Russia: A phenomenological study. *Health Education Research, 18*, 135–144.

Bennett, G. G., Wolin, K. Y., Viswanath, K., Askew, S., Puleo, E., & Emmons, K. M. (2006). Television viewing and pedometer-determined physical activity among multiethnic residents of low-income housing, *American Journal of Public Health, 96*, 1681–1685.

Bennett, J. A., & Flaherty-Robb, M. K. (2003). Issues affecting the health of older citizens: Meeting the challenge. *The Online Journal of Issues in Nursing, 8.* Retrieved October 3, 2007, from www.nursingworld.org/MainMenuCategories/ OJIN/TableofContentsVolume820 03/Num2May312003/CarePlanningforBaby Boomers.aspx.

Bephage, G. (2006). Meeting the healthcare needs of older homeless people. *Nursing Times, 102*, 38–41.

Berger, E. (2005, May 10). Study shows Alzheimer's may strike Latinos at an earlier age. *Houston Chronical*, p. 8.

Berridge, V. (2004). Historical and policy approaches. In M. Thorogood & Y. Coombes (Eds.), *Evaluating health promotion practice and methods* (pp. 11–26). New York: Oxford University Press.

Best, A., Stokols, D., Green, L. W., Leischow, S., Holmes, B., & Bucholtz, K. (2003). An integrative framework for community partnering to translate theory into effective health promotion strategy. *American Journal of Health promotion, 18*, 168–176.

Bickmore, T. W., Caruso, L., & Clough-Gorr, K. (2005). *Acceptance and usability of a relational interface by urban older adults.* Boston: Boston University School of Medicine.

Biegel, D. E., & Leibbrandt, S. (2006). Elders living in poverty. In B. Berkman & S. D'Ambruoso (Eds.), *Handbook of social work in health and aging* (pp. 167–180). New York: Oxford University Press.

Binstock, R. H. (2006–07). Older people and political engagement: From avid voters to "cooled-out" marks. *Generations, 30*, 24–30.

Birds, bees and HIV for seniors. (2007, August 17). *Toronto Star*, p. AA08.

Birkhead, G. S., Riser, M. H., Mesier, K., Tailon, T. C., & Klein, S. J. (2006). Youth development is a public health approach. *Journal of Public Health Management Practice*, November (Suppl), S1–S3.

Blankenship, K. M., Friedman, S. R., Dworkin, S., & Mantell, J. E. (2006). Structural interventions: Concepts, challenges and opportunities for research. *Journal of Urban Health, 83*, 59–72.

Blow, F. C., Bartels, S. J., Brockmann, L. M., & Van Citters, A. D. (2006). *Evidence-based practices for preventing substance abuse and mental health problems in older adults.* Rockville, MD: Older Americans Substance Abuse & Mental Health Technical Assistance Center.

Blow, F. C., Walton, M. A., Barry, K. L., Coyne, J. C., Mudd, S. A., & Copeland, L. A. (2000). The relationship between alcohol problems and health functioning of older adults in primary care settings. *Journal of the American Geriatrics Society, 45,* 769–774.

Blustein, J., & Fleischman, A. R. (2004). Urban bioethics: Adapting bioethics to the urban context. *Academic Medicine, 79,* 1198–1202.

Boerner, K., & Reinhardt, J. P. (2003). Giving while in need: Support provided by disabled older adults. *The Journals of Gerontology Series B: Psychological Sciences and Social Sciences, 58,* S297–S304.

Bonomi, A. E., Anderson, M. L., Reid, R. J., Carrell, D., Fishman, P. A., Rivara, F. P., et al. (2007). Intimate partner violence in older women. *The Gerontologist, 47,* 34–41.

Bopp, M., Lattimore, D., Wilcox, S., Laken, M., McClorin, L., Swinton, R., et al. (2007). Understanding physical activity participation in members of an African American church: A qualitative study. *Health Education Research, 22,* 815–826.

Borzi, P. (2007, February 21). Bringing back the six-on-six game: Granny Basketball offers nostalgic, yet gentle, physical activity. *New York Times,* p. C23.

Bottomley, J. A., Bissonette, A., & Snekvik, V. C. (2001). The lives of homeless older adults: Please, tell them who I am. *Geriatric Rehabilitation, 16,* 50–64.

Boutilier, M., Cleverly, S., & Labonte, R. (2000). Community as a setting for health promotion. In B. Poland, L. Green, & I. Rootman (Eds.), *Settings for health promotion: Linking theory and practice* (pp. 250–307). Newbury Park, CA: Sage.

Breslow, L. (2000). The social context of disease prevention and wellness promotion. In M. S. Jamner & D. Stokols (Eds.), *Promoting human wellness: New frontiers for research, practice, and policy* (pp. 38–77). Berkeley: University of California Press.

Brewer, C. (2004). *Doorway thoughts: Cross-cultural health care for older adults.* Sudbury, MA: Jones & Bartlett.

Brody, J. E. (2007, November 29). When the twilight years become unbearable. *New York Times,* p. 10.

Brounstein, P. J., Gardner, S. E., & Backer, T. (2006). Research to practice: Efforts to bring effective prevention to every community. *Journal of Primary Prevention, 27,* 91–109.

Brown, D. R., & Sankar, A. (1998). HIV/AIDS and aging minority populations. *Research on Aging, 20,* 865–884.

Brown, G. (2002, June). HIV/AIDS among older persons: A growing problem. *Minority Nurse Newsletter,* p. 1.

Brown, P. (2007). *Toxic exposures.* New York: Columbia University Press.

Brown, W. M., Consedine, N. A., & Magai, C. (2005). Altruism relates to health in an ethnically diverse sample of older adults. *Journals of Gerontology Series B: Psychological Sciences and Social Sciences, 60B,* 143–152.

Browne, C. (1995). Empowerment in social work practice with older women. *Social Work, 40,* 358–364.

Brucker, J. (2001). Walking a mile in their shoes: Sociocultural considerations in elder homelessness. *Geriatric Rehabilitation, 16,* 15–27.

Brush, S. B. (1996). Whose knowledge, whose genes, whose rights? In S. B. Brush & D. Stabinsky (Eds.), *Valuing knowledge: Indigenous people and intellectual rights* (pp. 1–31). Washington, DC: Island Press.

Bryant, L. L., Altpeter, M., & Whitclaw, N. A. (2006). Evaluation of health promotion programs for older adults: An introduction. *Journal of Applied Gerontology*, 25, 197–213.

Buchanan, D. R. (2000). *An ethic for health promotion: Rethinking the sources of human well-being*. New York: Oxford University Press.

———. (2006). Further reflections on a new ethic for health promotion. *Health Education & Behavior*, 33, 308.

Buckley, J. (2002). Holism and a health-promoting approach to palliative care. *International Journal of Palliative Nursing*, 8, 505–508.

Budrys, G. (2003). *Unequal health: How inequality contributes to health or illness*. New York: Rowman & Littlefield.

Buijs, R., Ross-Kerr, J., O'Brien, S., & Wilson, D. (2003). Promoting participation: Evaluation of a health promotion program for low income seniors. *Journal of Community Health Nursing*, 20, 93–107.

Bulatao, R. A., & Anderson, N. B. (Eds.). (2004). *Understanding racial and ethnic differences in health in late life: A research agenda*. Washington, DC: National Academies Press.

Bullock, K. (2006). Promoting advance directives among African Americans: A faith-based model. *Journal of Palliative Medicine*, 9, 183–195.

Bullock, K., & McGraw, S. A. (2006). A community capacity-enhancement approach to breast and cervical cancer screening among older women of color. *Health & Social Work*, 31, 16–25.

Bunde-Birouste, A. W. (2002). *Health promotion effectiveness: An analysis of the work at the XVIIth World Conference on Health Promotion and Health Education*. New York: World Health Organization.

Bunton, R., & Macdonald, G. (2002a). Introduction. In R. Bunton & G. Macdonald (Eds.), *Health promotion: Disciplines, diversity and developments* (2nd ed., pp. 1–8). London: Routledge.

Burbank, P. (Ed.). (2006). *Vulnerable older adults: Health care needs and interventions*. New York: Springer.

Bureau estimates number of children and adults in the states and Puerto Rico. (2005, March 10). *U.S. Census Bureau News*.

Burgener, S. C. (2004). *Prevalence of chronic disease in an inner city, minority older adult population*. Urbana: University of Illinois.

Burgess, J. (2006). Participatory action research. *Action Research*, 4, 419–437.

Burnett, P., & Matlins, A. (2006). *Civic engagement*. Paper prepared for the Blaine House Conference on Aging. Orono, ME: The University of Maine Center on Aging.

Burton, L. M. (1999). *Determinants of physical activity initiation and maintenance among community-dwelling older persons*. Retrieved July 2, 2007, from www.sciencedirect.com/science?_ob=MImg&_imagekey=B6WPG-45FJWCW-2K-1&_cdi=6990&_user=489277&_orig=search&_coverDate=11%2F30%2F1999& sk=999709994& view=c&wchp=dGLzVzz- zSkzS&md5=5f057c71bd5a415e01ead03eac001a87&ie =/sdarticle.pdf

Burton, L. M., & Whitfield, K. E. (2003). "Weathering" towards poorer health in later life: Co-morbidity in urban low-income families. *Public Policy & Aging Report*, 13, 13–18.

Burton, N. W., Turrell, G., & Oldenburg, B. (2003). Participation in recreational physical activity: Why do socioeconomic groups differ? *Health Education & Behavior, 30*, 225–244.

Butler, S. S. (2006). Older gays, lesbians, bisexuals, and transgendered persons. In B. Berkman & S. D'Ambruoso (Eds.), *Handbook of social work in health and aging* (pp. 273–281). New York: Oxford University Press.

Callahan, D., & Jennings, B. (2002). Ethics and public health: Forging a strong relationship. *American Journal of Public Health, 92*, 169–176.

Cameron, J. (2006, July 17). Fast facts: Civic engagement and older Americans—volunteerism. In *Fact Sheet*. Washington, DC: National Governors Association.

Carlton-LeNey, I. (2006–07). "Doing the Lord's work": African American elders' civic engagement. *Generations, 30*, 47–50.

Carr, D. B., Duchek, J. M., Meuser, T. M., & Morris, J. C. (2006). Older adult drivers with cognitive impairment. *American Family Physician, 73*, 1029–1038.

Carr, D. B., Flood, K., Steger-May, M., Schechtman, K. B., & Binder, E. F. (2006). Characteristics of frail older drivers. *Journal of the American Geriatric Society, 54*, 1125–1129

Carry, B. (2007, August 23). Many found sexually active into the 70s. *New York Times*, p. A15.

Carson, A. J., Chappell, N. L. & Knight, C. J. (2007). Promoting health and innovative health promotion practice through a community arts centre. *Health Promotion Practice, 8*, 366–374.

Castiel, L. D. (2003). Self care and consumer health. Do we need a public health ethics? *Journal of Epidemiology and Community Health, 57*, 5–6.

Castro, F. G., Elder, J., Coe, K., Tafoya-Barraza, H. M., Moratto, S., Campbell, N., et al. (1995). Mobilizing churches for health promotion in Latino communities: Companeros en la salud. *Journal of the National Cancer Institute Monograph, 18*, 127–135.

Catford, J. (2004). Health promotion's record card: How principled are we 20 years on? *Health Promotion International, 19*, 1–4.

Cattan, M. (2001). Practical health promotion: What have we learnt so far? In D. Chivas & A. F. Stears (Eds.), *Promoting the health of older people: The next step in health generation* (pp. 11–22). Buckingham, England: Open University Press.

Cattan, M., & Tilford, S. (2006). *Mental health promotion: A lifespan approach*. London, England: McGraw-Hill.

Center for Social Gerontology. (2001). *Fact sheet on tobacco & older persons*. Ann Arbor: University of Michigan.

Center for the Advancement of Health. (2006). *A new vision of aging: Helping older adults make healthier choices*. Washington, DC: Author.

Center on an Aging Society. (2003). *Obesity among older Americans: At risk for chronic conditions*. (Challenges for the 21st Century: Chronic and Disabling Conditions, Data Profile No. 10, pp. 1–5). Georgetown University.

———. (2004). *Cultural competence in health care: Is it important for people with chronic conditions?* (Challenges for the 21st Century: Chronic and Disabling Conditions, Data Profile No. 5, pp. 1–8). Georgetown University.

Centers for Disease Control and Prevention. (2001). Eliminate disparities in diabetes. Atlanta, GA: Author.

———. (2005, December 1). *Healthy aging for older adults.* Retrieved May 12, 2006, from www.cdc.gov/aging/.

———. (2006a). National Center for Injury Prevention and Control. Web-based injury statistics query and reporting system (WISQARS) [online]. Retrieved August 9, 2007, from www.cdc.gov/ncipc/wisqars.

———. (2006b). *Disaster planning goal: Protecting vulnerable older adults.* Atlanta, GA: Author.

———. (2007a). *Falls among older adults: An overview.* Retrieved August 9, 2007, from www.cdc.gov/ncipc/factsheet/adultfalls.htm.

———. (2007b). *Older adult drivers: Fact sheet.* Retrieved October 17, 2007, from www.cdc.gov/ncipe/factsheets/older.htm.

———. (2007c). *Eliminate disparities in diabetes.* Retrieved October 24, 2007, from www.cdc.gov/omh/AMH/factsheets/diabetes.htm.

Chapin, R., & Cox, E. O. (2001). Changing the paradigm: Strengths-based and empowerment-oriented social work with frail elders. *Journal of Gerontological Social Work, 36,* 165–179.

Chapin, R., Nelson-Becker, H., Gordon, T., & Terrebonne, S. (2002). *Aging and gay, lesbian, bisexual and transgendered older person.* Unpublished manuscript, University of Kansas School of Social Welfare.

Chapman, N. J., & Pancoast, D. L. (1985). Working with informal helping networks of the elderly: The experiences of three programs. *The Journal of Social issues, 41,* 47–65.

Chappell, N., Funk, L., Carson, A., MacKenzie, P., & Stanwick, R. (2006). Multi-level community health promotion: How can we make it work? *Community Development Journal, 41,* 352–366.

Charlesworth, G. (2000). Older adults who reported strain when caring for a spouse with disabilities had increased morality. *Evidence-Based Mental Health, 15,* 282.

Chen, H., Cheal, K., Herr, E. C. M., Zubritsky, C., & Levkoff, S. E. (2007). Religious participation as a predictor of mental health status and treatment outcomes in older persons. *International Journal of Geriatric Psychiatry, 22,* 144–153.

Cherniack, E. P., Senzel, R. S., & Pan, C. X. (2001). Correlates of use of alternative medicine by the elderly in an urban population. *The Journal of Alternative and Complementary Medicine, 7,* 277–280.

Chernoff, R. (2001a). Nutrition and health promotion in older adults. *The Journals of Gerontology Series A: Biological Sciences and Medical Sciences, 56,* 47–53.

———. (2001b). Nutrition. In E. A. Swanson, T. Tripp-Reimer, & K. Buckwalter (Eds.), *Health promotion and disease prevention in the older adult: Interventions and recommendations* (pp. 43–55). New York: Springer.

Chiriboga, D. A. (2004). Some thoughts on the measurement of acculturation among Mexican American elders. *Hispanic Journal of Behavioral Sciences, 28,* 274–292.

Chivas, D., & Stears, A. F. (Eds.). (2001). *Promoting the health of older people: The next step in health generation.* Buckingham, England: Open University Press.

Choi, H. (2007). *How do older adult volunteer instructors describe their peer teaching experiences at a Lifelong Learning Institute (LLI).* Unpublished manuscript, Pennsylvania State University.

Choi, N. G. (2005). *Assessment of depression needs of low-income older adults: Informal caregivers' and social service providers' perspectives.* Austin: Center for Social Work Research, University of Texas School of Social Work.

Choi, N. G., Burr, J. A., Mutchler, J. E., & Caro, F. G. (2007). Formal and informal volunteer activity: Spousal caregiving among older adults. *Research on Aging, 29,* 99–124.

Chu, L. D., & Kraus, J. F. (2004). Predicting fatal assault among the elderly using the National Incident-Based Reporting System Crime Data. *Homicide Studies, 8,* 71–95.

Chwalisz, K. (2003). Evidence-based practice: A framework for twenty-first-century scientist-practitioner training. *The Counseling Psychologist, 31,* 497–528.

Clark, A. P., Stuifbergen, A., Gottlieb, N. H., Voelmeck, W., Darby, D., & Delvilla, C. (2006). Health promotion in heart failure—a paradigm shift. *Holistic Nurse Practice, 20,* 73–79.

Clark, C. M., DeCarli, C., Mungas, D., Chui, H. I., Higdon, R., Nunez, J., et al. (2005). Earlier onset of Alzheimer Disease symptoms in Latino individuals compared to Anglo individuals. *Archives of Neurology, 62,* 774–778.

Clark, D. O., & Nothwehr, F. (1999). Exercise self-efficacy and its correlates among socioeconomically diverse older adults. *Health Education & Behavior, 26,* 535–546.

Clark, R. (2004). Significance of perceived racism: Toward understanding ethnic group disparities in health, the later years. In N. B. Anderson, R. A. Bulatao, & B. Cohen (Eds.), *Critical perspectives on racial and ethnic differences in health in late life* (pp. 540–566). Washington, DC: National Academies Press.

Classen, S., Garvin, C. W., Awadzi, K., Sundaram, S., Winter, S., Lopez, E. D. S., et al. (2006). Systematic literature review and models for older driver safety. *Topics in Geriatric Rehabilitation, 22,* 87–98.

Cleak, H., & Howe, J. L. (2003). Social network and use of social supports of minority elders in East Harlem. *Social Work in Health Care, 38,* 19–38.

Clevenger, C. K., & Quinn, M. E. (2007). *Primary prevention of Alzheimer's disease: Evaluation of a modified brain health promotion program in a continuing care retirement community.* Paper presented at the annual meeting of the American Public Health Association, Washington, DC.

Clift, S., & Morrissey, M. (2001). Health and the older traveler: Issues for health promotion. In A. Chiva & D. Stears (Eds.), *Promoting the health of older people* (pp. 132–143). Buckingham, England. Open University Press.

Cnaan, R. A., Boddie, S. C., & Kang, J. L. (2005). Religious congregations as social service providers for older adults. *Journal of Gerontological Social Work, 45,* 105–130.

Cohen, C. I., Sokolvsky, J., & Crane, M. (2001). Aging, homelessness, and the law. *Internacional Journal of Law and Psychiatry, 24,* 1–15.

Cohen, D., & Hale, J. (2002). Using economics in health promotion. In R. Bunton & G. Macdonald (Eds.), *Health promotion: Disciplines, diversity and developments* (2nd ed., pp. 178–196). London: Routledge.

Cohen, L., Perales, D. P., & Steadman, C. (2005). The O word: Why the focus on obesity is harmful to community health. *California Journal of Health Promotion*, *3*, 134–161.

Cohen, R. J., Kirsten, E., & Pan, C. X. (2002). Complementary and alternative medicine (CAM) use by older adults: A comparison of self-report and physician chart documentation. *The Journals of Gerontology Series A: Biological Sciences and Medical Sciences*, *57*, M223–M227.

Cohen-Mansfield, J., Marx, M. S., Biddison, J. R., & Guralnik, J. M. (2004). Socio-environmental exercise preferentes among older adults. *Preventive Medicine*, *38*, 804–811.

Collins, C. C., & Benedict, J. (2006). Evaluation of a community-based health promotion program for the elderly: Lessons from Seniors CAN. *American Journal of Health Promotion*, *21*, 45–48.

Collins, J. L., Giles, W., & Holmes-Chavez. (2007). Old dilemmas, new commitments: Toward a 21st century strategy for community health promotion. *Prevention of Chronic Diseases*, *4*, A42.

Collins, P. A., & Hayes, M. V. (2007). Twenty years since Ottawa and Epp: Researchers' reflections on challenges, gains and future prospects for reducing health inequalities in Canada. *Health Promotion International*, *22*, 337–345.

Committee on Population. (2004a). Critical Perspectives on *Racial and ethnic differences in health in late life*. Retrieved July 2, 2007, from www.nap.edu/openbook .php?isbn=0309092116.

———. (2004b). Understanding *Racial and ethnic differences in health in late life*: A research agenda. Retrieved July 2, 2007, from books.nap.edu/openbookphp?isbn =0309092477.

Connell, C. M. (1999). Older adults in health education research: Some recommendations. *Health Education Research*, *14*, 427–431.

Cook, K. E. (2007). Using critical ethnography to explore issues in health promotion. *Qualitative Health Research*, *15*, 129–138.

Coon, D. W., Lipman, P. D., & Ory, M. G. (2003). Designing effective HIV/AIDS social and behavioral interventions for the population of those age 50 and older. *Journal of Acquired Immune Deficiency Syndrome*, *33*, S194–S205.

Corburn, J. (2007). Reconnecting with our roots: American urban planning and public health in the twenty-first century. *Urban Affaire Review*, *42*, 688–713.

Cornisa, F., & Ghosh, R. (2006). The necessary contradictions of "community-led" health promotion: A case study of HIV prevention in an Indian red light district. *Social Science & Medicine*, *64*, 496–507.

Cortes, T., Lee, A., Boal, J., Mion, L., & Butler, A. (2004). Using focus groups to identify asthma care and education issues for elderly urban-dwelling minority individuals. *Applied Nursing Research*, *17*, 207–212.

Cottrell, R. R., Girvan, J. T., & McKenzie, J. F. (2002). *Principles & foundations of health promotion and education* (2nd ed.). San Francisco: Benjamin Cummings.

Coughlin, S. S. (2006a). Ethical issues in epidemiologic research and public health practice. *Emerging Themes in Epidemiology*, *3*, 16–22.

———. (2006b). Hope, ethics, and public health. *Journal of Epidemiology and Community Health*, *60*, 826–827.

Cousins, S. O. (2003). A self-reference thinking model: How older adults may talk themselves out of being physically active. *Health Promotion Practice, 4,* 439–448.

Crane, M., Bryne, K., Fu, R., Lipmann, B., Mirabelli, F., Rota-Bartelink, A., et al. (2005). The causes of homelessness in later life: Findings from a 3-nation study. *Journals of Geronology Series B: Psychological Sciences and Social Sciences, 60,* 153–159.

Crane, M., & Warnes, A. M. (2001). Older people and homelessness: Prevalence and causes. *Topics in Geriatric Rehabilitation, 16,* 1–14.

Cribb, A., & Duncan, P. (2002). Introducing ethics into health promotion. In R. Bunton & G. Macdonald (Eds.), *Health promotion: Disciplines, diversity and developments* (2nd ed., pp. 271–283). London: Routledge.

Crowley, M. (2003). *Generation X speaks out on civil engagement and the decennial census: An ethnographic approach.* Washington, DC: U.S. Census Bureau.

Crystal, S., Akincigil. A., Sambamoorthi, U., Wenger, N., Fleishman, J. A., Zingmond, D. S., et al. (2003). The diverse older HIV-positive population: A national profile of economic circumstances, social support, and quality of life. *Journal of Acquired Immune Deficiency Syndrome, 33,* S76–S83.

Cullinane, P. (2006–07). Promoting purposeful lives for greater good: Civic engagement programs of aging organizations. *Generations, 30,* 109–111.

Cunningham, G. O., & Michael, Y. L. (2004). Concepts guiding the study of the impact of the built environment on physical activity for older adults: A review of the literature. *American Journal of Health Promotion, 12,* 435–443.

Curry, L., & Jackson, J. (2003). The science of including older ethnic and racial group participants in health-related research. *The Gerontologist, 43,* 15–17.

Damron-Rodríguez, J., Frank, J. C., Enríquez-Haass, V. L., & Reuben, D. B. (2005). Definitions of health among diverse groups of elders: Implications for health promotion. *Public Health & Aging, 29,* 11–16.

Dancy, J., & Ralston, P. A. (2002). Health promotion and black elders. *Research on Aging,* 24, 218–242.

Daniels, N. (2001). Justice, health, and healthcare. *The American Journal of Bioethics,* 1, 2–16.

D'Augelli, A. R., & Grossman, A. H. (2001). Disclosure of sexual orientation, victimization, and mental health among lesbian, gay, and bisexual older adults. *Journal of Interpersonal Violence, 16,* 1008–1027.

Davies, M. (2001). Health promotion and sexuality in later life. In A. Chiva & D. Stears (Eds.), *Promoting the health of older people* (pp. 86–98). Buckingham, England: Open University Press.

Davis, K. (2006). What is effective intervention?—using theories of health promotion. *British Journal of Nursing, 15,* 252–256.

Davis, L. A., & Chesbro, S. B. (2003). Integrating health promotion, patient education, and adult education principles with the older adult: A perspective for rehabilitation professionals. *Journal of Allied Health, 32,* 106–109.

Davis, M. P., & Srivastava, M. (2003). Demographics, assessment and management of pain in the elderly. *Drugs & Aging, 20,* 23–57.

Davison, J. A., Moreno, P. R., Badimon, J. J., Lopez-Candales, A., Giachello, A. L. M., Ovalle, F., et al. (2007). Cadiovascular disease prevention and care in Latino and Hispanic subjects. *Endocrinology Practice, 13,* 77–85.

DeCoster, V. A., & George, L. (2005). An empowerment approach to elders living with diabetes: A pilot study of a community-based self-help group—the Diabetes Club. *Educational Gerontology, 31*, 699–713.

DeHaven, M. J., Hunter, I. B., Wilder, L., Walton, J. W., & Berry, J. (2004). Health programs in faith-based organizations: Are they effective? *American Journal of Public Health, 94*, 1030–1036.

De La Rue, M., & Coulson, I. (2003). The meaning of health and well-being: Voices from older rural women. *Rural & Remote Health, 3*, 192.

Delgado, M. (1977). Puerto Rican spiritualism and the social work profession. *Social Casework, 58*, 451–458.

———. (1979). Herbal medicine in the Puerto Rican community. *Health and Social Work, 4*, 24–40.

———. (1995). Puerto Rican elders and natural support systems: Implications for human services. *Journal of Gerontological Social Work, 24*, 115–129.

———. (1996a). Aging research and the Puerto Rican community: The use of an elder advisory committee of intended respondents. *The Gerontologist, 36*, 406–408.

———. (1996). Puerto Rican food establishments as social service organizations: Results of an asset assessment. *Journal of Community Practice, 3*, 57–70.

———. (1997a). Interpretation of Puerto Rican elder research findings: A community forum of research respondents. *Journal of Applied Gerontology, 16*, 317–332.

———. (1997b). Role of Latina-owned beauty parlors in a Latino community. *Social Work, 42*, 445–453.

———. (1998). Puerto Rican elders and merchant establishments: Natural caregiving systems or simply businesses? *Journal of Gerontological Social Work, 30*, 33–45.

———. (1999). *Social work practice in nontraditional urban settings.* New York: Oxford University Press.

———. (2000). *Community social work practice within an urban context: The potential of a capacity enhancement perspective.* New York: Oxford University Press.

———. (2006). *Designs and methods for youth-led research.* Thousand Oaks, CA: Sage.

———. (2007). *Social work practice with Latinos: A cultural assets paradigm.* New York: Oxford University Press.

Delgado, M., Jones, K., Rohani, M. (2004). *Social work practice with refugee and immigrant youth in the United States.* Boston: Allyn & Bacon.

Delgado, M., & Staples, L. (2008). *Youth-led community organizing: Theory and action.* New York: Oxford University Press.

Delgado, M., & Zhou, H. (2008). *Youth-led urban health promotion: A community capacity enhancement approach.* New York: Aronson.

Desai, R. A., Maciejewski, P. K., Dausey, D. J., Caldarone, B. J., & Potenza, M. N. (2004). Health correlates of recreational gambling in older adults. *American Journal of Psychaitry, 161*, 1672–1679.

Deutsch, C. (2007, October 23). For love and a little money. *New York Times*, pp. H1, H4.

Dickson, R. A. (2006, December 6). Arts program takes seniors beyond bingo. *Florida Times-Union* (Jacksonville), p. 3.

Diczfalusy, E. (1996). The third age, the Third World and the third millennium. *Contraception, 53,* 1–7.

Diehr, P., & Patrick, D. L. (2003). Trajectories of health for older adults over time: Accounting fully for death. *Annals of Internal Medicine, 139,* 416–420.

Dietz, T. L., & Wright, J. D. (2005a). Victimization of the elderly homeless. *Case Management Journal, 6,* 15–21.

———. (2005b). Age and gender differences and predictors of victimization of the older homeless. *Journal of Elder Abuse and Neglect, 17,* 37–60.

Dill, A., Brown, P., Clambrone, D., & Rakowski, W. (1990). The meaning and practice of self-care by older adults. *Research on Aging, 17,* 8–41.

Djousse, L., Biggs, M. L., Mukamal, K. J., & Siscovick, D. S. (2007). Alcohol consumption and Type 2 diabetes among older adults: The Cardiovascular Health Study. *Obesity, 16,* 1758–1765.

Donahue, P., & McDonald, L. (2005). Gay and lesbian aging: Current perspectives and future directions for social work practice and research. *Families in Society, 86,* 359–366.

Dornelas, E., Stepnowski, R., Fischer, E., & Thompson, P. (2007). Urban ethnic minority women's attendance at health clinic vs. church based exercise programs. *Journal of Cross-Cultural Gerontology, 27,* 129–136.

Dorsett, B. M. (2004). Cultural competence and health literacy: Making your health promotion program accessible to diverse groups of older adults. *Live Well, Live long: Health Promotion and Disease Prevention for Older Adults* (Issue Brief 4), 1–6.

Doty, M. M., & Holmgren, A. L. (2005). *Health care disconnect: Gaps in coverage and care for minority adults: Findings from the Commonwealth Fund Biennial Health Insurance Survey (2005).* New York: The Commonwealth Fund.

Downes, T., & Channer, K. S. (2001). Plight of elderly people who are made homeless in hospital. *British Medical Journal, 323,* 229.

Drum, C. E., Krahn, G., Culley, C., & Hammond, L. (2005). Recognizing and responding to the health disparities of people with disabilities. *California Journal of Health Promotion, 3,* 29–42.

Duan, N. Fox, S., Derose, K. P., Carson, S., & Stockdale, S. (2005). Identifying churches for community-based mammography promotion: Lessons from the LAMP Study. *Health Education & Behavior, 32,* 536–548.

Duffy, D., Goldberg, J., & Buchwald, D. (2006). Using mail to reach patients seen at an urban health care facility. *Journal of Health Care for the Poor and Underserved, 17,* 522–531.

Duggleby, W., & Raudonis, B. M. (2006). Dispelling myths about palliative care and older adults. *Seminal Oncology Nursing, 22,* 58–64.

Duncan, P. (2004). Dispute, dissent and the place of health promotion in a "disrupted tradition" of health improvement. *Public Understanding of Science, 13,* 177–199.

Dunkle, R. E., & Jeon, H. S. (2006). The oldest old. In B. Berkman & S. D'Ambruoso (Eds.), *Handbook of social work in health and aging* (pp. 191–204). New York: Oxford University Press.

Dunn, K. S., & Riley-Doucet, C. K. (2007). Self-care activities captured through discussion among community-dwelling older adults. *Journal of Holistic Nursing, 25,* 160–169.

Duxbury, A. (2000). Disease prevention versus health promotion: Pitfalls of preventive care in the geriatric population. In M. S. Jamner & D. Stokols (Eds.), *Promoting human wellness: New frontiers for research, practice, and policy* (pp. 398–423). Berkeley: University of California Press.

Easom, L. R. (2003). Concepts in health promotion. Perceived self-efficacy and barriers in older adults. *Journal of Gerontological Nursing, 29,* 11–19.

Eccleston, M., & Priestman, S. (2007). *Leading with experience: Engaging older adults as community leaders.* Washington, DC: Experience Corps National Office.

Edmondson, R. (2005). Wisdom in later life: Ethnographic approaches. *Ageing & Society, 25,* 339–356.

Eisner, M. D., Yelin, E. H., Katz, P. P., Shiboski, S. C., Henke, J., & Blanc, P. D. (2000). Predictors of cigarette cessation among adults with asthma. *American Journal of Public Health, 90,* 1307–1311.

Elena, S. H. Y., Chen, E. H., Kim, K. K., & Abdulrahim, S. (2002). Smoking among Chinese Americans: Behavior, knowledge, and beliefs. *American Journal of Public Health, 92,* 1007–1013.

Elliot, V. S. (2001, August 6). Cultural competency critical in elder care. *AM/News.* Retrieved May 18, 2005, from www.ama-assn.org/amednews/2001/08/06/hll20806htm.

Emlet, C. A. (Ed.). (2004a). *HIV/AIDS and older adults: Challenges for individuals, families, and communities.* New York: Springer.

Emlet, C. A. (2004b). Knowledge and use of AIDS and aging services by older, HIV- infected adults. In C. C. Poindexter & S. Keigher (Eds.), *Midlife and older adults and HIV: Implications for social service research, practice, and policy* (pp. 9–24). New York: Haworth Press.

Emlet, C. A., & Poindexter, C. (2004). Underserved, unseen, and unheard: Integrating programs for HIV-infected and HIV-affected older adults. *Health & Social Work, 29,* 86–96.

Endres, T. (2005). Research shows non-profit organizations unprepared to use older volunteers. Retrieved June 6, 2007, from www.ncoa.org/content/cfm?sectionalD=65anddetail=1000.

Endres, T., & Holmes, C. A. (2006–07). Respectability in America: Guiding principles for civic engagement among adults 55-plus. *Generations, 30,* 101–108.

Englander, F., Hodson, T. J., & Terregrossa, R. A. (1996). Economic dimensions of slip and fall injuries. *Journal of Forensic Science, 41,* 733–746.

Environmental Protection Agency. (2007, September 19). *Environmental fact sheet for older adults available in 11 languages.* Washington, DC: Author.

Erben, R., Franzkowiak, P., & Wenzel, E. (2000). People empowerment vs. social capital: From health promotion to social marketing. *Health Promotion Journal of Australia, 9,* 179–182.

Espino, D. V., & Oakes, L. (2007). Access issues in the care of Mexican-origin elders. In J. L. Angel & K. E. Whitfield (Eds.), *The health of aging Hispanics: The Mexican-origin population* (pp. 195–201). New York: Springer.

Evans, G. W., Kantrowitz, E., & Eshelman, P. (2002). Housing quality and psychological well-being among the elderly population. *The Journals of Gerontology Series B: Psychological Sciences and Social Sciences, 57,* P381–P383.

Evans, W. D., Renaud, J. M., Finkelstein, E., Kamerow, D. B., & Brown, D. S. (2006). Changing perceptions of the childhood obesity epidemic. *American Journal of Health Behavior, 30,* 167–176.

Evidence in health promotion: An international challenge and opportunity. (2003). *Harvard Health Policy Review, 4,* 1–3.

Faison, W. E., & Mintzer, J. E. (2005). The growing, ethnically diverse aging population: Is our field advancing with it? *American Journal of Geriatric Psychiatry, 13,* 541–544.

Falk, L. W., Sobal, J., Bisogni, C. A., Connors, M., & Devine, C. M. (2001). Managing healthy eating: Definitions, classifications, and strategies. *Health Education & Behavior, 28,* 425–439.

Ferraro, K. F. (2006). Imagining the disciplinary advancement of gerontology: Whither the tipping point. *The Gerontologist, 46,* 571–573.

Fetterman, D. M. (2003). Youth and evaluation: Empowerment social change agents. In K. Sabo (Ed.), *Youth participatory evaluation: A field in the making* (pp. 89–92). San Francisco: Jossey-Bass.

Finch, B. K., Hummer, R. A., Reindi, M., & Vega, W. A. (2002). Validity of self-rated health among Latino(a)s. *American Journal of Epidemiology, 155,* 755–759.

Finkelstein, E. A., Chen, H., Miller, T. R., Corso, P. S., & Stevens, J. A. (2005). A comparison of the case-control and case-crossover designs for estimating medical costs of non-fatal fall-related injuries among older Americans. *Medical Care, 43,* 1087–1091.

Finkelstein, R., & Netherland, J. (2005). Sexual minority groups and urban health. In S. Galea & D. Vlahov (Eds.), *Handbook of urban health* (pp. 79–102). New York: Springer.

Firdaus, M., Mathew, M. K., & Wright, J. (2006). Health promotion in older adults: The role of lifestyle in the metabolic syndrome. *Geriatrics, 61,* 18–22, 24–25.

Fischer, F. (2003). *Citizens, experts, and the environment: The politics of local knowledge.* Durham, NC: Duke University Press.

———. (2004). Professional expertise in a deliberative democracy. *The Good Society, 13,* 21–27.

Flegal, K. M., Williamson, D. F., Pamuk, E. R., & Rosenberg, H. M. (2004). Estimating deaths attributable to obesity in the United States. *American Journal of Public Health, 94,* 1486–1489.

Fleischman, A. R., & Barondess, J. A. (2004). Urban health: A look out our windows. *Academic Medicine, 79,* 1130–1132.

Flood, M., & Newman, A. M. (2007). Obesity in older adults: Synthesis of findings and recommendations for clinical practice. *Journal of Gerontological Nursing, 33,* 19–35.

Foley, D. J., Heimovitz, H. K., Guralnik, J. M., & Brock, D. B. (2002). Driving life expectancy of persons aged 70 years and older in the United States. *American Journal of Public Health, 92,* 1284–1289.

Fong, C. (2006). *Testimony for the roundtable discussion on the reauthorization of the Older Americans Act.* February 14, 2006. Senate Health, Education, Labor, and Pensions Committee. Washington, DC.

Ford, A. F. (2000). *Older black women, health, and the black helping experience.* Pittsburgh, PA: University of Pittsburgh School of Social Work.

Foster-Cox, S. C., Mangadu, T., Jacquez, B., & Corona, A. (2007). The effectiveness of the *promotora* (community health worker) model of intervention for improving pesticide safety in US/Mexico border homes. *California Journal of Health Promotion, 5,* 62–75.

Fountain, H. (2006, January 15). On not wanting to know what hurts you. *New York Times,* p. 14.

Francoeur, R., & Elkins, J. (2006). Older adults with diabetes and complications. In B. Berkman & S. D'Ambruoso (Eds.), *Handbook of social work in health and aging* (pp. 29–39). New York: Oxford University Press.

Freedman, M. (1999). *How Baby Boomers will revolutionize retirement and transform America.* New York: Public Affairs.

———. (2006–07). The social purpose encore career: Baby boomers, civic engagement, and the next stage of work. *Generations, 30,* 43–46.

Freeman, E. F., Gange, S. J., Munoz, B., & West, S. K. (2006). Driving status and risk of entry into long-term care in older adults. *American Journal of Public Health, 96,* 1254–1259.

Freudenberg, N. (2004). Community capacity for environmental health promotion: Determinants and implications for practice. *Health Education & Behavior, 31,* 472–490.

———. (2007). From lifestyle to social determinants: New directions for community health promotion research and practice. *Preventing Chronic Disease, 4,* 1–2.

Fried, L. P. (2000). *Health promotion for older adults: What is the potential?* Eleventh Annual Herbert Lourie Memorial Lecture on Health Policy. Syracuse, NY: University of Syracuse.

Fried, L. P., Carlson, M. C., Freedman, M., Frick, K. D., Glass, T. A., Hill, J., et al. (2006). A social model for health promotion for an aging population: Initial evidence on the Experience Corps Model. *Journal of Urban Health, 81,* 64–78.

Friedman, D., & Parekh, R. (2007). Obesity, depression, and health promotion for older African American adults. Paper presented at the American Public Health Association Annual Meeting, November 8, 2007, Washington, DC.

Fritsch, T. (2005). HIV/AIDS and the older adult: An exploratory study of the age-related differences in access to medical and social services. *Journal of Applied Gerontology, 24,* 35–54.

Fronstin, P. (2005). Employee Benefit Research Institute sources of health insurance and characteristics of the uninsured: Analysis of the March 2005 Current Population Survey. EBRI Issue Brief 287, 1–31. Retrieved July 2, 2007, from www .ebri.org/publications/ib/index.cfm?fa=ibDisp&content_id=3597.

Fung, A. (2004). *Empowerment participation: Reinventing urban democracy.* Princeton, NJ: Princeton University Press.

Fusco, C. (2007). "Healthification" and the promises of space. *International Review for the Sociology of Sport, 41,* 43–63.

Fustes, O. (2002). *Diabetic cooking for Latinos.* Washington, DC: American Diabetic Association.

Fuzhong, L., Fisher, K. J., Harmer, P., & McAuley, E. (2005). Falls self-efficacy as a mediator of fear of falling in an exercise intervention for older adults. *The Journals of Gerontology Series B: Psychological Sciences and Social Sciences, 60,* P34–P40.

Galea, S., & Vlahov, D. (2005). Urban health: Evidence, challenges, and directions. *Annual Review of Public Health, 26,* 341–365.

Gallagher, E. M. (1985). Capitalize on elder strengths. *Journal of Gerontological Nursing, 11,* 13–17.

Gallagher, E. M., & Beecher, P. (1987). Health promotion in prisons: An adjunct to the pill parade. *Canadian Journal of Public Health, 78,* 95–97.

Gallagher, S., & Povey, R. (2006). Determinants of older adults' intentions to vaccinate against influenza: A theoretical application. *Journal of Public Health, 28,* 139–144.

Galloway, R. D. (2003). Health promotion: Causes, beliefs and measurements. *Clinical Medicine & Research, 1,* 249–258.

Galston, W. A., & Lopez, M. H. (2006). Civic engagement in the United States. In L. B. Wilson & S. P. Simson (Eds.), *Civic engagement and the baby boomer generation: Research, policy, and practice perspectives* (pp. 3–19). New York: Haworth Press.

Galvez, M. P., Morland, K., Raines, C., Kobil, J., Siskind, J., Godbold, J., et al. (2007). Race and food store availability in an inner-city neighborhood. *Public Health Nutrition, 11,* 624–631

Gamble, V. N. (1997). Under the shadow of Tuskegee: African Americans and health care. *American Journal of Public Health, 87,* 1773–1778.

Gardner, J. (1988). *The experience corps.* Retrieved September 21, 2007, from www .experiencecorps.org/about_us/gardners_vision.html.

Garfield, S. A., Malozowski, S., Chin, M. H., Narayan, K. M. V., Glasgow, R. E., Green, L. W., et al. (2003). Considerations for diabetes translational research in real-world settings. *Diabetes Care, 26,* 2670–2674.

Garibaldi, B., Conde-Martel, A., & O'Toole, T. P. (2005). Self-reported comorbidities, perceptive needs, and sources for usual care for older and younger homeless adults. *Journal of General Internal Medicine, 20,* 726–730.

Garrett, N., & Martini, E. M. (2007). The boomers are coming: A total costs of care model of the impact of population aging on the cost of chronic conditions in the United States. *Disease Management, 27,* 51–60.

Garroutte, E. M., Sarkisian, N., Arguelles, L., Goldberg, J., & Buchwald, D. (2006). Cultural identities and perceptions of health among health care providers and older American Indians. *Journal of General Internal Medicine, 21,* 111–116.

Gearin, E., & Kahle, C. (2006). Teen and adult perceptions of urban green space Los Angeles. *Children, Youth and Environments, 16,* 25–48.

Gelfand, D. E. (2003). *Aging and ethnicity: Knowledge and services* (2nd ed.). New York: Springer.

Geronurse Online. (2006). *Ethnogeriatrics and cultural competence for nursing practice.* Retrieved September 24, 2007, from www.consultgerirn.org/topics/ ethnogeriatrics_and_cultural_competence_for_nursing.

Gfroerer, J., Penne, M., Pemberton, M., & Folsom, R. (2003). Substance abuse treatment among older adults in 2020: The impact of the aging baby-boom cohort. *Drug and Alcohol Dependence, 69,* 127–135.

Ghent University. (2007). Setting an ethical agenda for health promotion. Retrieved September 12, 2007, from www.healthpromotionethics.eu/.

Ginn, J., Arber, S. & Cooper, H. (2001). Inequalities in health-related behaviour among older people. In D. Chivas & A. F. Stears (Eds.), *Promoting the health of older people: The next step in health generation* (pp. 23–39). Buckingham, England: Open University Press.

Ginsberg, B. R. (2001). How education empowers older adults. *Activities, Adaptation & Aging, 25,* 1–11.

Given, B. A., & Given, C. W. (2001). Health promotion for older adults in a managed care environment. In E. A. Swanson, T. Tripp-Reimer, & K. Buckwalter (Eds.), *Health promotion and disease prevention in the older adult: Interventions and recommendations* (pp. 219–241). New York: Springer.

Glanz, K., Lewis, F. M., & Rimer, B. K. (1997). The scope of health promotion and Education. In K. Glanz, F. M. Lewis, & B. K. Rimer (Eds.), *Health behavior and health education: Theory, research, and practice* (2nd ed., pp. 3–18). San Francisco: Jossey-Bass.

Glasgow, R. E., Lichtenstein, E., & Marcus, A. C. (2003). Why don't we see more translation of health promotion research to practice? Rethinking the efficacy-to-effectiveness transition. *American Journal of Public Health, 93,* 1261–1267.

Goetzel, R. Z. (2007). Can health promotion programs save Medicare money? *Clinical Interventions in Aging, 2,* 117–122.

Gold et al. (2006) *Race/ethnicity, socioeconomic status, and lifetime morbidity burden in the Women's Health Initiative: A cross-sectional analysis.* Retrieved July 2, 2007, from www.liebertonline.com/doi/pdf/10.1089/jwh.2006.15.1161.

Goldman, R., Hunt, M. K., Allen, J. D., Hauser, S., Maeda, M., & Sorensen, G. (2003). The life history interview method: Applications to intervention development. *Health Education & Behavior, 30,* 564–581.

Gomperts, J. S. (2006–07). Toward a bold new policy agenda: Five ideas to advance civic engagement opportunities for older Americans. *Generations, 30,* 85–89.

Gonyea, J. (2002). Age through ethnic lenses: Caring for the elderly in a multicultural society (review). *Journal of Health Politics, Policy and Law, 27,* 863–865.

Gonyea, J., & Googins, B. K. (2006–07). Expanding the boundaries of corporate volunteerism: Tapping the skills, talents, and energy of retires. *Generations, 30,* 78–84.

Gonzalez, D. (2005, January 25). Paying a price for doughnuts, burgers and pizza. *New York Times,* p. A25.

Gonzalez, H. M., Haan, M. N., & Hinton, L. (2001). Acculturation and the prevalence of depression in older Mexican Americans: Baseline results of the Sacramento area study on aging. *Journal of the American Geriatric Society, 49,* 498.

Goodkin, K., Heckman, T., Siegel, K., Linsk, N., Khamis, I., Lee, D., et al. (2003). "Putting a face" on HIV infection/AIDS in older adults: A psychosocial context. *Journal of Acquired Immune Deficiency Syndrome, 33,* S171–S184.

Goodroad, B. K. (2003). HIV and AIDS in people older than 50: A continuing concern. *Journal of Gerontological Nursing, 29,* 18–24.

Goodstadt, M. (2007). *Community development & organization.* Toronto, Ontario, Canada: Centre for Health Promotion, University of Toronto.

Gordon, C. (2004). Cultural approaches to promoting activity for older adults, *Journal on Active Aging,* November–December, 22–28.

Granville, G. (2001). Intergenerational health promotion and active citizenship. In A. Chiva & D. Stears (Eds.), *Promoting the health of older people* (pp. 40–51). Buckingham, England: Open University Press.

Gray, M. J., & Acierno, R. (2002). Symptom presentations of older adult crime victims: description of a clinical sample. *Journal of Anxiety Disorders, 16,* 299–309.

Green, B. L., Lewis, R. K., Wang, M. Q., Pearson, S., & Rivers, B. (2004). Powerlessness, destiny, and control: The influence on health behaviors of American Americans. *Journal of Community Health, 29,* 15–27.

Green, J. (2000). The role of theory in evidence-based health promotion practice. *Health Education Research, 15,* 125–129.

Green, J., & Tones, K. (1999). For debate. Towards a secure evidence base for health promotion. *Journal of Public Health Medicine, 21,* 133–139.

Green, L., Nathan, R., & Mercer, S. (2001). The health of health promotion in public policy: Drawing inspiration from the tobacco control movement. *Health Promotion Journal of Australia, 11,* 20–29.

Greene, R., & Cohen, H. L. (2005). Social work with older adults and their families: Changing practice paradigms. *Families in Society, 86,* 367–374.

Greenfield, E. A., & Marks, N. F. (2004). Formal volunteering as a protective factor for older adults' psychological well-being. *The Journals of Gerontology: Series B: Psychological Sciences and Social Sciences, 59B,* S258–S264.

Greenwald, H. P., & Beery, W. L. (2001). Reducing isolation among inner-city elders: An outcome evaluation. *Health Promotion Practice, 2,* 233–241.

Greve, F. (2008, July 20). More seniors finding love, skipping remarriage. *Lawrence Journal-World* (Kansas), p. 6A.

Gross, J. (2007, October 9). Aging and gay, and facing prejudice in twilight. *New York Times,* pp. A1, A25.

———. (2008a, March 6). New generation gap emerges as older addicts seek help. *New York Times,* A1, A20.

———. (2008b, March 25). Its appeal slipping, the senior center steps livelier. *New York Times,* p. A14.

Gruman, J. C. (2004) *Health promotion for older adults: Nice or necessary?* Paper presented at the American Geriatric Society Confronting Ageism and Economics in Promoting Elder Health, November 23.

Grundy, K., & Holt, G. (2001). The socioeconomic status of older adults: How should we measure it in studies of health inequalities? *Journal of Epidemiology of Community Health, 55,* 895–904.

Guralnick, S. (2003). Promoting health for ethnic older adults. *Northwest Geriatric Education Center Viewpoint, 12,* 1–2.

Gurnack, A. M. (Ed.). (1999). *Older adults' misuse of alcohol, medicines, and other drugs: Research and practice issues.* New York: Springer.

Haber, D. (2007). *Health promotion and aging: Implications for the health profession* (4th ed.). New York: Springer.

Haber, D., & Looney, C. (2003). Health promotion directory: Development, distribution, and utilization. *Health Promotion Practice, 4,* 72–77.

Hahn, J. A., Kushel, M. B., Bangsberg, D. R., Riley, E., & Moss, A. R. (2006). The aging of the homeless population: Fourteen year trends in San Francisco. *Journal of General Internal Medicine, 21,* 775–778.

Hajjar, I., Frost, B., Lacy, J. E., & Kotchen, J. (2006). Association of primary care providers health habits with lifestyle counseling to hypertensive elderly patient: Results of a national survey. *California Journal of Health Promotion, 4,* 114–122.

Hammond, E., & Treisman, G. J. (2007, December 1). HIV and psychiatric illness. Special report: Comorbidity. *Psychiatric Times,* p. 57.

Harris, A. H. S. & Thoresen, C. E. (2005). Volunteering is associated with delayed mortality in older people: Analysis of the Longitudinal Study of Aging. *Journal of Health Psychology, 10,* 730–752.

Harris, G. (2006, February 24). Urban dance pilot puts new spring in older adults' steps. *University of Calgary in the News,* pp. 1–2.

Harris, Y., & Cooper, J. K. (2006). Depressive symptoms in older people predict nursing home admission. *Journal of the American Geriatrics Society, 54,* 593–597.

Hartman-Stein, P., & Potkanowicz, E. (2003). Behavioral determinants of healthy aging: Good news for the baby boomer generation. *The Online Journal of Issues in Nursing, 8,* www.nursingworld.org/MainMenuCategories/OJIN/Tableof ContentsVolume82003/Num2May312003/CarePlanningforBabyBoomers .aspx). Accessed October 3, 2007.

Hartocollis, A. (2008, July 18). Rise seen in medical efforts to improve very long lives. *New York Times,* pp. A1, C12.

Harvard School of Public Health. (2004). *Reinventing aging: Baby boomers and civic engagement.* Boston: Author.

Hatchett, B. F. (1999). Alcohol problems among older African-American women. *Journal of Religion and Health, 38,* 149–154.

Hawe, P., & Shiell, A. (2000). Social capital and health promotion: A review. *Social Science & Medicine, 51,* 871–885.

Hawthorne, F. (2007, October 23). Greater obstacles to retirement for women. *New York Times,* p. H13.

Hayward, M. D., Warner, D. F., & Crimmins, E. M. (2007). Does longer life mean better health? Not for native-born Mexican-Americans in the Health and Retirement Survey. In J. L. Angel & K. E. Whitfield (Eds.), *The health of aging Hispanics: The Mexican-origin population* (pp. 85–95). New York: Springer.

Health Promotion Agency. (2007). *Health promotion theories and models.* Belfast, Northern Ireland: Author. Retrieved November 9, 2007, from www.health promotionagency.org.uk/Healthpromotion/Health/section5.htm.

Health Resources and Services Administration. (2003). *Homeless and elderly: Understanding the special health needs of elderly persons who are homeless.* Washington, DC: Author.

Health Watch. (2002). African Americans and older adults and HIV/AIDS. Retrrieved May 25, 2006, from www.hwatch.org/hivseniors.html.

Healthy messages: How to attract today's older adult. (2003, March/April). *Journal of Active Aging,* pp. 26–32.

Heller, L. (2007, May 8). Latino food guide promotes healthy eating. *Food Navigator USA.Com.* Retrieved November 6, 2007, from www.foodnavigator-usa .com/news/printNewsBis.asp?id=76359.

Helwig, D. (2006, November 5). Urban planning influences physical activity, public health. *SooToday.com,* 1–5. Retrieved September 21, 2007, from http://www .spptoday.com/content/newsfull_story.asp?StoryNumber=20671.

Henderson, K. A., & Ainsworth, B. E. (2000). Sociocultural perspectives on physical activity in the lives of older African American and American Indian women: A cross cultural activity participation study. *Women Health, 31*, 1–20.

———. (2003). A synthesis of perceptions about physical activity among older African American and American Indian women. *American Journal of Public Health, 93*, 313–317.

Hendricks, C. S., Hendricks, D. L., Webb, S. J., Davis, J. B., & Spencer-Morgan, B. (2005). Fostering self-efficacy as an ethical mandate in health promotion practice and research. *OnLine Journal of Health Ethics.* Retrieved August 28, 2007, from ethicsjournal.umc.edu/ojs2/indexphp/ojhe/article/viewPDFIntersitial/18/25.

Henkin, N., & Zapf, J. (2006–07). How communities can promote civic engagement of people age 50-plus. *Generations, 30*, 72–77.

Henry J. Kaiser Family Foundation. (2005). *Profile of African Americans, Latinos, and whites with Medicare: Implications for outreach efforts for the new drug benefit.* Menlo Park, CA: Henry J. Kaiser Family Foundation.

Herr, K., & Decker, S. (2004). Older adults with severe cognitive impairment: Assessment of pain. *Annals of Long-Term Care: Clinical and Aging, 12*, 46–52.

Hertzman, C. (2004). The life-course contribution to ethnic disparities in health. In N. B. Anderson, R. A. Bulatao, & B. Cohen (Eds.), *Critical perspectives on racial and ethnic differences in health in late life* (pp. 145–170). Washington, DC: National Academies Press.

Hess, P. L., Reingold, J. S., Jones, J., Fellman, M. A., Knowles, P., Ravenell, J. E., et al. (2007). Barbershops as hypertension detection, referral, and follow-up centers for black men. *Hypertension, 49*, 1040–1046.

Heumann, L. F., McCall, M. E. & Boldy, D. P. (2000). *Empowering frail elderly people: Opportunities and impediments in housing, health, and support service delivery.* Westport, CT: Greenwood Publishers.

Heynen, N. C., & Lindsey, G. (2003). Correlates of urban forest canopy cover: Implications for local public works. *Public Works Management & Policy, 8*, 33–47.

Heynen, N. C., Perkins, H. A., & Roy, P. (2006). The political ecology of uneven urban space. *Urban Affairs Review, 42*, 3–25.

Hickey, A. M. (2006). *The "graying" of an epidemic: Social policy, health promotion, and HIV/AIDS education and prevention for adults over 50 in the Midwest, theoretical findings.* Paper presented at the annual meeting of the American Sociological Association, Montreal, August 2006.

Higgins, J. W., Naylor, P. J., & Day, M. (2008). Seed funding for health promotion: Sowing sustainability or skepticism? *Community Development Journal, 43*, 210–221

Hill, F. J. (2003). Towards a new model for health promotion: An analysis of complementary and alternative medicine and models of health promotion. *Health Education Journal, 62*, 369–380.

Himes, C. L. (2002). Elderly Americans. *Population Bulletin, 56*, 1–40.

Hinterlong, J., McBride, A. M., Tang, F., & Danso, K. (2006). Issues in elder service and volunteerism worldwide: Toward a research agenda. In L. B. Wilson & S. P. Simson (Eds.), *Civic engagement and the baby boomer generation: Research, policy, and practice perspectives* (pp. 213–246). New York: Haworth Press.

Hinterlong, J. E., & Williamson, A. (2006–07). The effects of civic engagement on current and future cohorts of older adults. *Generations, 30*, 10–17.

Hirschhorn, L. (1979). Alternative service and the crisis of the professions. In J. Case & R. C. R. Taylor (Eds.), *Co-ops, communes, and collectives: Experiments in social change in the 1960s and 1970s* (pp. 153–193). New York: Pantheon.

Ho, E. E., Waltz, J., Ramstack, J., Homoki, J., Kligman, E., Meredith, K., et al. (1987). Health peers: A delivery model for health promotion among the elderly. *Educational Gerontology, 13*, 427–436.

Hodes, R. J. (2006). *A new vision of aging: Helping older adults make healthier choices.* Washington, DC: Center for the Advancement of Health.

Holder, B. (2001). Interventions with elderly African American diabetics. In E. A. Swanson, T. Tripp-Reimer, & K. Buckwalter (Eds.), *Health promotion and disease prevention in the older adult: Interventions and recommendations* (pp. 203–218). New York: Springer.

Holmes, P. (2006). Supporting older people: Promoting falls prevention. *British Journal of Community Nursing, 11*, 247–248, 250.

Holstein, M. (2006). A critical reflection on civic engagement. *Public Policy & Aging Report, 16*, 1, 21–26.

Hooker, S. P., Cirilli, L., & Wicks, L. (2007). Walkable neighborhoods for seniors: Alameda County experience. *Journal of Applied Gerontology, 26*, 157–181.

Hosay, C. K. (2003). Long-term care and before: Current perspective roles for health educators working with older people. *Health Promotion Practice, 4*, 457–463.

Howze, E. H., Baldwin, G. T., & Kegler, M. C. (2004). Environmental health promotion: Bridging traditional environmental health and health promotion. *Health Education & Behavior, 31*, 429–440.

Hsueh, M. N., & Yeh, M. L. (2006). A conceptual analysis of the process of empowering the elderly at the community level. *Hu Li Za Zhi, 53*, 5–10.

Huang, C. H., Chen, S. W., Yu, Y., Chen, P. R., & Lin, Y. C. (2002). The effectiveness of health promotion education programs for community elderly. *Journal of Nursing Research, 10*, 261–270.

Hudson, R. B. (2006). Terms of engagement: The right and left look at elder civic activism. *Public Policy & Aging Report, 16*, 13–18.

Hudson, R. B. (2006–07). Aging in a public space: The roles and functions of civic engagement. *Generations, 30*, 51–58.

Hui, E. R., & Rubenstein, L. Z. (2006). Promoting physical activity band exercise in older adults. *Journal of the American Medical Directors Association, 7*, 310–314.

Hummer, R. A., Benjamins, M. B., & Rogers, R. G. (2004). Racial and ethnic disparities in health and mortality among U.S. elderly population. In N. B. Anderson, R. A. Bulatao, & B. Cohen (Eds.), *Critical perspectives on racial and ethnic differences in health in late life* (pp. 53–94). Washington, DC: National Academies Press.

Hurworth, R., Harvey, G., & Rutter, A. (2002, October/November). *Empowering older adults through engagement in the evaluation process: Examples from adult and community education projects in Victoria.* Paper presented at the Australasian Evaluation Society International Conference, Wollongoing, Australia.

Hwang, S. W., O'Connell, J. J., Lebow, J. M., Bierer, M. F., Orav, E. J., & Brennan, T. A. (2001). Health care utilization among homeless adults prior to death. *Journal of Health Care for the Poor and Underserved, 21,* 50–58.

Idler, E. (2006, October). *Religiousness and spirituality as community resources for aged persons with chronic illness.* Paper presented at Taking Community Action Against Pain: Translating Research on Chronic Pain among Older Adults, Cornell Institute for Translational Research, New York.

Inelman, E. M., Gasparini, G., & Enzi, G. (2005). HIV/AIDS in older adults: A case report and literature review. *Geriatrics, 60,* 26–30.

Jackson, J. S., & Knight, K. M. (2006). Race and self-regulatory health behaviors: The role of the stress response and the HPA Axis in physical and mental health disparities. In K. Warner Schaie & L. L. Carstensen (Eds.), *Social structures, aging, and self-regulation in the elderly* (pp. 189–207). New York: Springer.

Jackson, N., & Waters, E. (2005). Criteria for the systematic review of health promotion and public health interventions. *Health Promotion International, 20,* 367–374.

Jamner, M. S. (2000). Introduction: New frontiers for research, practice, and policy. In M. S. Jamner & D. Stokols (Eds.), *Promoting human wellness: New frontiers for research, practice, and policy* (pp. 1–15). Berkeley: University of California Press.

Jamner, M. S., & Stolois, D. (Eds.). (2000). *Promoting human wellness: New frontiers for research, practice, and policy.* Berkeley: University of California Press.

Jang, Y., Borenstein, A. R., Chiriboga, D. A., Phillips, K., & Mortimer, J. A. (2006). Religiosity, adherence to traditional culture, and psychological well-being among African American elders. *Journal of Applied Gerontology, 25,* 343–355.

Jasinski, J. L., & Dietz, T. L. (2003). Domestic violence and stalking among older adults: An assessment of risk factors. *Journal of Elder Abuse & Neglect, 15,* 3–18.

Jennings-Sanders, A. (2003). Using health fairs to examine health promotion behaviors of older African Americans. *The Association of Black Nursing Faculty Journal, 14,* 1–14.

John A. Hartford Foundation. (2005). *Helping older adults adopt healthy habits: Agencies find evidence-based programming gets results.* New York: Author.

Johnson, B. (2006, May 15). The not-so-skinny: U.S. population weighs in as the world's most obese; America home to nearly 23% of planet's excessively overweight individuals. *American Demographics, 43.*

Johnson, C., Parel, M., Cobb, M., & Uy, D. (2003). *The strength of the infrastructure of volunteer agencies and its capacity to absorb "baby boomer" volunteers.* Boston: Harvard-Metlife Foundation.

Johnson, J. E. (2000). Assessment of older urban drivers by nurse practitioners. *Journal of Community Health Nursing, 17,* 107–114.

Johnson, R. W., & Schaner, S. G. (2005). Value of unpaid activities by older Americans tops $160 billion per year. *Perspectives on Productive Aging, 4,* 1–5.

Johnson, R. W., & Wiener, J. M. (2006). *A profile of frail older Americans and their caregivers.* Washington, DC: Urban Institute.

Jones, D. R. (2005). Older adults: A secret weapon in the war against poverty. *CSS (Community Service Society) News, 21,* 1–4.

Jones, S. C., & Donovan, R. J. (2004). Does theory inform practice in health promotion in Australia? *Health Education Research, 19,* 1–14.

Joyce, G. F., Goldman, D. P., Leibowitz, A. A., Alpert, A., & Bao, Y. (2005). A socioeconomic profile of older adults with HIV. *Journal of Health Care for the Poor and Underserved, 16*, 19–28.

Kahan, B., & Goodstadt, M. (2001). The interactive domain model of best practices in health promotion: Developing and implementing a best practices approach to health promotion. *Health Promotion Practice, 2*, 43–67.

Kai, R., Klein, R. S., Schoenbaum, E. E., Anastos, K., Minkoff, H., & Sacks, H. S. (2006). Aging and HIV infection. *Journal of Urban Health: Bulletin of the New York Academy of Medicine, 83*, 31–42.

Kakabadse, N. K., & Kakabadse, A. (2003). Developing reflective practitioners through collaborative inquiry: A case study of the UK Civic Service. *International Review of Administrative Sciences, 69*, 365–383.

Kales, H. C., & Mellow, A. M. (2006) Race and depression: Does race affect the diagnosis and treatment of late-life depression? *Geriatrics, 61*, 18–21.

Karuza, J. (2001). Immunizations. In E. A. Swanson, T. Tripp-Reimer, & K. Buckwalter (Eds.), *Health promotion and disease prevention in the older adult: Interventions and recommendations* (pp. 179–202). New York: Springer.

Katula, J. A., Sipe, M., Rejeski, W. J., & Focht, B. C. (2006). Strength training in older adults: An empowering intervention. *Medical Science & Sports Exercise, 38*, 106–111.

Kaushik, V. P., Snih, S. A., Ray, L. A., Raji, M. A., Markides, K. S., & Goodwin, J. S. (2007). Factors associated with seven-year incidence of diabetes complications among older Mexican Americans. *Gerontology: International Journal of Experimental Clinical and Behavorial Gerontology, 53*, 194–199.

Keigher, S. M., Stevens, P. E., & Plach, S. K. (2004). Midlife women with HIV: Health, social, and economic factors shaping their futures. In C. C. Poindexter & S. Keigher (Eds.), *Midlife and older adults and HIV: Implications for social service research, practice, and policy* (pp. 43–58). New York: Haworth Press.

Keller, C., & Fleury, J. (1999). *Health promotion for the elderly*. Thousand Oaks, CA: Sage.

Kelley-Moore, J. A., & Ferraro, K., F. (2004). The black/white disability gap: Persistent inequality in later life. *Journals of Gerontology: Series B: Psychological Sciences and Social Sciences, 59B*, S34–S43.

Kennedy, D. (2004). The role of a facilitator in a community of philosophy inquiry. *Metaphilosophy, 35*, 744–765.

Kessell, E. R., Bhatia, R., Bamberger, J. D., & Kushel, M. B. (2006). Public health care utilization in a cohort of homeless adult applicants to a supportive housing program. *Journal of Urban Health, 83*, 860–873.

Kickbusch, I., McCann, W., & Sherbon, T. (2008). Adelaide revisited: From healthy public policy to health in all policies. *Health Promotion International, 23*, 1–4.

Kim, H., & Lee, J. (2006). Unequal effects of elders' health problems on wealth across race and ethnicity. *Journal of Consumer Affairs, 39*, 148–172.

Kim, H., & Richardson, V. E. (2006). Driving cessation and consumption expenses in the later years. *The Journals of Gerontology Series B: Psychological and Social Sciences, 61*, S347–S353.

King, S. V., Burgess, E. D., Akinyela, M., Courts-Spriggs, M., & Parker, N. (2005). "Your body is God's temple": The spiritualization of health beliefs in multigenerational African-American families. *Research on Aging, 27*, 420–446.

Kittles, R. A., Santos, E. R., Oji-Njideka, N., & Bonilla, C. (2007). Race, skin, color and genetic ancestry: Implications for biomedical research on health disparities. *California Journal of Health Promotion, 5*, 9–23.

Kiyak, H. A., & Reichman, M. (2005). Barriers to and enablers of older adults' use of dental services. *Journal of Dental Education, 69*, 976–986.

Klein, R. S., Schoenbaum, E. E., Anastos, K., Minkoff, H., Sacks, H. S., & Kohli, R. (2006). Aging and HIV infection. *Journal of Urban Health: Bulletin of the New York Academy of Medicine, 83*, 31–110.

Kleinfield, N. R. (2006a, January 9). Diabetes and its awful toll quietly emerge as a crisis: As cases surge in New York, so do fears of an overburdened medical system. *New York Times*, pp. A1, A18.

———. (2006b, January 10). Living at an epicenter of diabetes, defiance and despair. *New York Times*, pp. A1, A20.

Klinedinst, N. J. (2005). Effects of a nutrition education program for urban, low-income, older adults: A collaborative program among nurses and nursing students. *Journal of Community Health Nursing, 22*, 93–104.

Koch, T., Mann, S., Kralik, D., & van Loon, A. M. (2005). Reflection. *Journal of Research in Nursing, 10*, 261–278.

Koch, T., Selim, P., & Kral, K. D. (2002). Enhancing lives through the development of a community-based participatory action research programs. *Journal of Clinical Nursing, 11*, 109–117.

Kochtitzky, C. S., Frumkin, H., Rodriguez, R., Dannenberg, A. L., Rayman, J., Rose, K., et al. (2006, December 22). Urban planning and public health at CDC. *MMWR, 55*(SUP02), 34–38.

Koelen, M. A., Vaandrager, L., & Colomer, C. (2001). Health promotion research: Dilemmas and challenges. *Journal of Epidemiology & Community Health, 55*, 257–262.

Koenig, H. G. (2003). Health care and faith communities: How are they related? *Journal of General Internal Medicine, 18*, 962–963.

Kolata, G. (2007, January 3). Data on Hispanic immigrants presents puzzle on aging. *New York Times*, pp. A16.

Kolt, G. S., Oliver, M., Schofield, G. M., Kerse, N., Garrett, N., & Latham, N. K. (2006). An overview and process evaluation of TeleWalk: A telephone-based counseling intervention to encourage walking in older adults. *Health Promotion International, 21*, 201–208.

Koplan, J. P., & Livengood, J. R. (1994). The influence of changing demographic patterns on our health promotion priorities. *American Journal of Preventive Medicine, 10*, 42–44.

Korper, S. P., & Raskin, I. E. (2007). *Substance abuse by older adults: Estimates of future impact on the treatment system.* Rockville, MD: Office of Applied Studies, SAMHSA.

Kostis, J. B. (2004). Treatment of hypertension in older adults: An updated look at the role of calcium antagonists. *The American Journal of Geriatric Cardiology, 12*, 319–327.

Krause, N. (2004). Common facets of religion, unique facets of religion, and life satisfaction among older African Americans. *The Journals of Gerontology Series B: Psychological and Social Sciences, 59,* S109–S117.

Krause, N., Liang, J., Shaw, B. A., Sugisawa, H., Kim, H. K., & Sugihara, Y. (2002). Religion, death of a loved one, and hypertension among older adults in Japan. *The Journals of Gerontontology Series B: Psychological Sciences and Social Sciences, 56,* S96–S107.

Kreuter, M. W. (2005). Commentary on public health advocacy to change corporate practices. *Health Education & Behavior, 32,* 355–362.

Kreuter, M. W., Rosa, C. De, Howze, E. H., & Baldwin, G. T. (2004). Understanding wicked problems: A key to advancing environmental health promotion. *Health Education & Behavior, 31,* 441–454.

Krumeich, A., Weijts, W., Reddy, P., & Meijer-Weitz, A. (2001). The benefits of anthropological approaches for health promotion research and practice. *Health Education Research, 16,* 121–130.

Kuhlmann, R., & Ruddell, R. (2005). Elderly jail inmates: Problems, prevalence and public health. *California Journal of Health Promotion, 3,* 49–60.

Kuller, L. H. (2003). On reconsidering community-based health promotion. *American Journal of Public Health, 93,* 557–574.

Kuo, F. E., & Sullivan, W. C. (2001). Aggression and violence in the inner-city. *Environment and Behavior, 33,* 543–571.

Kutner, M., Greenberg, E., Jin, Y., & Paulsen, C. (2006). *The health literacy of America's adults: Results from the 2003 National Assessment of Adult Literacy.* Washington, DC: U.S. Department of Education.

Kweon, B. S., Sullivan, W. C., & Wiley, A. R. (1998). Green common spaces and the social integration of inner-city older adults. *Environment and Behavior, 30,* 832–858.

Lafreniere, S. (2004). Health promotion of the elderly: A conceptual matter. *Sente Publique, 16,* 303–312.

Lang, J. E., Lawry, D., & Anderson, L. (2005, October). *Implementing diverse national strategies to address health promotion in older adults.* Paper presented at the 3rd National Prevention Summit Innovations in Community Prevention, Washington, DC.

Lauder, W., Mummery, K., & Sharkey, S. (2006). Social capital, age and religiosity in people who are lonely. *Journal of Clinical Nursing, 15,* 334–340.

Lautenschalger, N. T., Almeida, O., Flicker, L., & Janca, A. (2004). Can physical activity improve the mental health of older adults? *Annals of General Hospital Psychiatry, 3,* 3–12.

LaVeist, T. A. (2006). Disentangling race and socioeconomic status: A key to understanding health inequalities. *Journal of Urban Health, 82*(iii), 26–34.

Laverack, G. (2004). *Health promotion practice: Building empowered communities.* Maidenhead, England: Open University Press.

Lee, M. M., Carpenter, B., & Meyers, L. S. (2006). Representations of older adults in television advertisements. *Journal of Aging Studies, 21,* 23–30.

Lee, S. Y. D., Gazmararian, J. A., Arozullah, A. M., & Brown, J. (2006). Health literacy and social support among elderly Medicare enrollees in a managed plan. *Journal of Applied Gerontology, 25,* 324–337.

Lee, T. C., Hanlon, J. G., & Ben-David, J. (2005). Risk factors for cardiovascular disease in homeless adults. *Circulation, 11,* 2629–2635.

Leibson, C. L., Toteson, A. N. A., Gabriel, S. E., Ransom, J. E., Melton, J. L. (2002). Mortality, disability, and nursing home use for persons with and without hip fracture: A population-based study. *Journal of the American Geriatrics Society, 50,* 1644–1650.

Lette, L., (2003). Enabling citizen participation of older adults through social and political environments. In L. Lette, P. Rigby, & D. Stewart (Eds.), *Using environments to enable occupational performance* (pp. 71–80). Thorofare, NJ: Slack Incorprated.

Levin, J., Chatters, L. M., & Taylor, R. J. (2005). Religion, health and medicine in African Americans: Implications for physicians. *Journal of the National Medical Association, 97,* 237–249.

Levin, L., & Ashton, J. R. (2006). It is necessary to distinguish between health promotion and promoting health. *Journal of Epidemiology and Community Health, 60,* 115.

Leviton, L. C., Snell, E., & McGinnis, M. (2000). Urban issues in health promotion strategies. *American Journal of Public Health, 90,* 863–866.

Levy, B. R., & Pilver, C. (2006). Commentary: The dynamic relationship between age stereotypes and wisdom in old age. In K. Warner Schaie & L. L. Carstensen (Eds.), *Social structures, aging, and self-regulation in the elderly* (pp. 55–67). New York: Springer.

Lewis, S. (2001, September). *Approaching the problem of defining "health" and "disease" from the perspectives of evolutionary psychology and Darwinian medicine.* Paper presented at the Joint Symposium of the Society for the Study of Human Biology and the Human Biological Association: The Changing face of Disease: Implications for Society. Cambridge, England.

Linder, J. F., & Meyers, F. J. (2007). Palliative care for prison inmates: "Don't let me die in prison." *Journal of the American Medical Association, 298,* 894–901.

Linnan, L. A., & Ferguson, Y. O. (2007). Beauty salons: A promising health promotion setting for reaching and promoting health among African American women. *Health Education & Behavior, 34,* 517–530.

Liss, P. E. (2000). Setting goals in health promotion: A conceptual and ethical platform. *Medicine, Health Care & Philosophy, 3,* 169–173.

Little, J. S., & Triest, R. K. (2001). *Seismic shifts: The economic impact of demographic change: An overview.* Boston: Federal Reserve Bank of Boston.

Lloyd, L. L., Ammary, N. J., Epstein, L. G., Johnson, R., & Rhee, K. (2006). A transdisciplinary approach to improve health literacy and reduce disabilities. *Health Promotion Practice, 7,* 331–335.

Lloyd, L. J. J., Epstein, L. G., Johnson, R., & Rhee, K. (2006). A transdisciplinary approach approach to improving health literacy and reducing disparities. *Health Promotion Practice, 7,* 331–335.

Lloyd-Jones, D. M., Evans, J. C., & Levy, D. (2005). Hypertension in adults across the age spectrum: Current outcomes and control in the community. *Journal of the American Medical Association, 294,* 466–472.

Locher, J. L., Ritchie, C. S., Roth, D. L., Baker, P. S., Bodner, E. V., & Allman, R. M. (2004). Social isolation, support, and capital and nutritional risk in an older sample: Ethnic and gender differences. *Social Science & Medicine, 60,* 747–761.

Loeb, S. J. (2006). African American older adults coping with chronic health conditions. *Journal of Transcultural Nursing, 17,* 139–147.

Loeb, S. J., & Staffensmeier, D. (2006). Older male prisoners: Health status, efficacy beliefs, and health-promotion behaviors. *Journal of Correctional Health Care, 12,* 269–278.

Loeb, S. J., Steffensmeier, D., & Lawrence, F. (2008). Comparing incarcerated and community-dwelling older men's health. *Western Journal of Nursing Research, 30,* 234–249.

Lopez, R. P. (2007). Neighborhood risk factors for obesity. *Obesity, 15,* 2111–2119.

Loprest, P., & Uccello, C. (1997). *Implications for changing Medicare eligibility.* New York: The Commonwealth Fund.

Love, A. S., & Love, R. J. (2007, February 1). Depression and diet in elderly community- dwelling Mexican and European Americans. *Psychiatric News,* pp. 1–4.

Luh, J. (2003). Ethnicity, older adults, and long-term care. *Innovations: Enhancing Ability in Dementia Care, 2,* 1–4.

Lum, T. Y., & Lightfoot, E. (2005). The effects of volunteering on the physical and mental health of older people. *Research on Aging, 27,* 31–55.

Lunenfeld, B. (2002). The ageing male: Demographics and challenges. *World Journal of Urology, 20,* 11–16.

Lyle, Y., & Kasi, E. (2002). Learning from the inquiry: Lessons for using collaborative inquiry as an adult learning strategy. *New Directions for Adult and Continuing Education, 94,* 93–104.

Lynde, B. (1992). Nutrition promotion for mature adults: A case study of peer education. *Journal of Nutrition for the Elderly, 11,* 19–31.

Macdonald, G., & Burton, R. (2002). Health promotion: Disciplinary development. In R. Bunton & G. Macdonald (Eds.), *Health promotion: Disciplines, diversity and developments* (2nd ed., pp. 9–28). London: Routledge.

MacDonald, T. H. (1998). *Rethinking health promotion: A global approach.* London: Routledge.

Mack, K. A., & Ory, M. G. (2003). AIDS and older Americans at the end of the twentieth century. *Journal of Acquired Immune Deficiency Syndromes, 33,* S131–S137.

MacLean, M. J. (2001). *Information sheet on HIV/AIDS and aging. Report for the Health Promotion and Programs Branch.* Ottawa: Health Canada.

Maddox, M. (1999). Older women and the meaning of health. *Journal of Gerontological Nursing, 25,* 26–33.

Mahoney, K. J., & Zooda, K. (2006). Approaches to empowering individuals and communities. In B. Berkman & S. D'Ambruoso (Eds.), *Handbook of social work in health and aging* (pp. 809–816). New York: Oxford University Press.

Mail, P. D., & Safford, L. (2003). LGBT disease prevention and health promotion: Wellness for gay, lesbian, bisexual, and transgender individuals and communities. *Clinical Research and Regulatory Affairs, 20,* 183–204.

Manning, T. T. (2006). Defining the relationships between civic engagement and leadership in later life. In L. B. Wilson & S. P. Simson (Eds.), *Civic engagement and the baby boomer generation: Research, policy, and practice perspectives* (pp. 171–192). New York: Haworth Press.

Marcus, M. B. (2006, July 31). "Graying" of HIV takes mental toll, too; depression levels 13 times higher in NYC study. *USA Today,* p. 6D.

Bibliography

Margen, S., & Lashof, J. C. (2000). Afterword. In M. S. Jamner & D. Stokols (Eds.), *Promoting human wellness: New frontiers for research, practice, and policy* (pp. 697–699). Berkeley: University of California Press.

Markey, S. (2003). *Older adults of color and environmental health. Listening sessions and interviews: To impact public policy and develop a national agenda on the environment and aging.* San Francisco: American Society on Aging.

Markides, K. S., Eschbach, K., Ray, L., & Peek, M. K. (2007). Census disability rates among older people by race/ethnicity and type of Hispanic origin. In J. L. Angel & K. E. Whitfield (Eds.), *The health of aging Hispanics: The Mexican-origin population* (pp. 165–180). New York: Springer.

Marks, R., & Allegrante, J. P. (2005). A review and synthesis of research for self-efficacy-enhancing interventions reducing chronic disability: Implications for health education practice (Part II). *Health Education Practice, 6,* 148–156.

Marks, R., & Shive, S. E. (2007). "Health for all": Ethical imperative or unattainable ideal? *Health Promotion Practice, 8,* 28–30.

Marshall, V. W., & Altpeter, M. (2005). Cultivating social work leadership in health promotion and aging: Strategies for active aging interventions. *Health and Social Work, 30,* 135–144.

Martinez, I. L., & Carter-Pokras, O. (2006). Assessing health concerns and barriers in a heterogeneous Latino community. *Journal of Health Care for the Poor and Underserved, 17,* 899–909.

Martinez, R. J. (1999). Close friends of God: An ethnographic study of health of older Hispanic adults. *Journal of Multicultural Nursing & Health, 5,* 40–45.

Martinson, M. (2006–07). Opportunities or obligations? Civic engagement and older adults. *Generations, 30,* 59–65.

Martinson, M., & Minkler, M. (2006). Civic engagement and older adults: A critical perspective. *The Gerontologist, 46,* 318–324.

Marzilli, T. S., Schuler, P. B., Willhoit, K. F., & Stepp, M. F. (2004). Effect of a community-based strength and flexibility program on performance-based measures of physical fitness in older African-American adults. *California Journal of Health Promotion, 2,* 92–98.

Mash, B., & Meulenburg-Buskens, J. (2001). "Holding it lightly": The cooperative inquiry group: A method for developing educational materials. *Medical Education, 35,* 1108–1114.

Massanari, R. M., Barth-Jones, D., Chapleski, E., Mahlmeister, L., & Smitherman, H. (2002). Mental health disparities in an elderly urban population. *Abstract of the Academy of Health Services Research & Health Policy Meeting, 19,* 29.

Maylahn, C., Alongi, S., Alongi, J., Moore, M. J., & Anderson, L. A. (2005). Data needs and uses for older adult health surveillance: Perspectives from state agencies. *Preventing Chronic Disease, 2.* Retrieved October 3, 2007, from www.pubmedcentral.nih.gov/articleerender.fegi?artid=1364511.

McBride, A. M. (2006–07). Civic engagement, older adults, and inclusion. *Generations, 30,* 66–71.

McBride, A. M., Sherraden, M. S., & Pritzer, S. (2006). Civic engagement among low-income and low-wealth families: In their words. *Family Relations, 55,* 152–162.

McCabe, B. W., Hertzog, M., Grasser, C. M., & Walker, S. N. (2005). Practice of health-promoting behavior by nursing home residents. *Western Journal of Nursing Research, 27,* 1000–1016.

McCabe-Sellers, B., & Johnston, R. (2006). Health promotion and disease prevention in the elderly. In R. Chernoff (Ed.), *Geriatric nutrition: The health professional's handbook* (pp. 519–557). Sudbury, MA: Jones & Bartlett, Inc.

McCarthy, M., Ruiz, E., Gale, B., Karam, C., & Moore, N. (2004). The meaning of health: Perspectives of Anglo and Latino older women. *Health Care for Women International, 25*, 950–969.

McCray, A. T. (2005). Promoting health literacy. *Journal of the American Medical Informatics Association, 12*, 152–163

McDonald-Miszczak, L., Wister, A. V., & Gutman, G. M. (2001). Predicting self-care among older adults with arthritis. *Journal of Aging and Health, 13*, 120–145.

McGinnis, J. M., Williams-Russo, P., & Knickman, J. R. (2002). The case for more active policy attention to health promotion. *Health Affairs: The Policy Journal of the Health Sphere, 21*, 78–93.

McKenzie, J. F., & Smeltzer, J. L. (2001). *Planning, implementing, and evaluating health program programs: A primer* (3rd ed.). Boston: Allyn & Bacon.

McKnight, J. L. (1994). Two tools for well-being: Health systems and communities. *American Journal of Preventive Medicine, 10*, 23–25.

McLeroy, K. R., Norton, B. L., Kegler, M. C., Burdine, J. N., & Sumaya, C. V. (2003). Community-based interventions. *American Journal of Public Health, 93*, 529–533.

McMullen, C. K., & Luborsky, M. R. (2006). Self-rated health appraisal as cultural and identity process: African American elders' health and evaluative rationales. *The Gerontologist, 48*, 431–438.

McNeill, T. (2006). Evidence-based practice in an age of relativism: Toward a model for practice. *Social Work, 51*, 147–156.

McQueen, D. V. (2000). Perspectives on health promotion: Theory, evidence, practice and the emergence of complexity. *Health Promotion International, 15*, 95–97.

McVittie, C., & Willock, J. (2006). "You can't fight windmills": How older men do health, ill health, and masculinities. *Qualitative Health Research, 16*, 788–801.

McWilliam, C. L., Stewart, M., Brown, J. B., McNair, S., Desai, K., Patterson, M., et al. (1997). Creating empowering meaning: An interactive process of promoting health with chronically ill older Canadians. *Health Promotion International, 12*, 111–123.

McWilliam, C. L., Stewart, M., Brown, J. B., McNair, S., Donner, A., Desai, K., et al. (1999). Home-based health promotion for chronically ill older persons: Results of a randomized controlled trial of a critical reflection approach. *Health Promotion International, 14*, 27–41.

Mendes de Leon, C. F., & Glass, T. A. (2004). The role of social and personal resources in ethnic disparities in late-life health. In N. B. Anderson, R. A. Bulatao, & B. Cohen (Eds.), *Critical perspectives on racial and ethnic differences in health in late life* (pp. 353–405). Washington, DC: National Academies Press.

Meecham, S. (2006). Prejudice undermines health promotion. *Nursing Standard, 20*, 32–33.

Meier, B. M., & Shelley, D. (2006). The fourth pillar of the Framework Convention on tobacco control: Harm reduction and the international human rights to health. *Public Health Reports, 121*, 494–500.

Menec, V. H., Shooshtari, S., & Lambert, P. (2007). Ethnic differences in self-rated health among older adults. *Journal of Aging & Health, 19*, 62–86.

Merzel, C., & D'Afflitti, J. (2003). Reconsidering community-based health promotion: Promise, performance, and potential. *American Journal of Public Health, 93*, 557–574.

Meyer, M. H., & Wilmouth, J. M. (2006). Changing demographics, stagnant social policies: An introduction, *Research on Aging, 28*, 265–268.

Middle-aged adults most likely to use complementary medicine. (2007, March 30). *Drug Week*, p. 44

Miller, A. M., & Iris, M. (2002). Health promotion attitudes and strategies in older adults. *Health Education & Behavior, 29*, 249–267.

Miller, C. A. (2003). *Nursing for wellness in older adults: Theory and practice.* Hagerstown, MD: Lippincott Williams & Wilkins.

Miller, K. K., & Dabson, B. (2005). *Age as asset: The contribution of youth and retirees to rural well-being.* St. Louis, MO: Center for Social Development, George Warren Brown School of Social Work, Washington University in St. Louis.

Milligan, S., Maryland, P., Ziegler, H., & Ward, A. (1987). Natural helpers as street health workers among the black urban elderly. *The Gerontologist, 27*, 712–715.

Min, J. W. (2005). Cultural competency: A key to effective social work with racially and ethnically diverse elders. *Families in Society, 86*, 347–358.

Minkler, M. (2000). Health promotion at the dawn of the 21st century: Challenges and dilemmas. In M. S. Jamner & D. Stokols (Eds.), *Promoting human wellness: New frontiers for research, practice, and policy* (pp. 349–377). Berkeley: University of California Press.

Minkler, M., & Checkoway, B. (1988). Ten principles for geriatric health promotion. *Health Promotion International, 3*, 277–285.

Minkler, M., Schauffler, H., & Clements-Nolle, K. (1999). Health promotion for older Americans in the 21st century. *American Journal of Health Promotion, 14*, 371–379.

Missouri Rural Health Association. (2006). *Senior health matters: Focus on health promotion.* Fact Sheet 8, pp. 1–3.

Mitchell, N., Wiener, J., & Gage, B. (2006). *Case studies of health promotion in the aging network: Division of Services for Aging and Adults with Physical Disabilities in Delaware.* Washington, DC: RTI International.

Mittelmark, M. B. (2008). Setting an ethical agenda for health promotion. *Health Promotion International, 23*, 78–85.

Montalto, C. P., Bhargava, V., & Hong, G. S. (2006). Use of complementary and alternative medicine by older adults: An exploratory study. *Complementary Health Practice Review, 11*, 27–46.

Moody-Ayers, S., Lindquist, K., Sen, S., & Covinsky, K. E. (2007). Childhood social and economic wellbeing and health in older age. *American Journal of Epidemiology, 166*, 1059–1067.

Moon, A., & Rhee, S. (2006). Immigrant and refugee elders. In B. Berkman & S. D'Ambruoso (Eds.), *Handbook of social work in health and aging* (pp. 205–217). New York: Oxford University Press.

Moreno-John, G., Gachie, A., Fleming, C. M., Napoles-Springer, A., Mutran, E., Manson, S. M., et al. (2004). Ethnic minority older adults participating in clinical research: Developing trust. *Journal of Aging and Health, 16*, 938–123S.

Morenoff, J. D., & Lynch, J. W. (2004). What makes a place healthy? Neighborhood influences on racial/ethnic disparities in health over the life course. In N. B. Anderson, R. A. Bulatao, & B. Cohen (Eds.), *Critical perspectives on racial and ethnic differences in health in late life* (pp. 406–449). Washington, DC: National Academies Press.

Morley, J. E. (2002). Drugs, aging, and the future [Editorial]. *The Journals of Gerontology Series A: Biological Sciences and Medical Sciences, 57*, M2–M6.

Morley, J. E., & Flaherty, J. H. (2002). It's never too late: Health promotion and illness prevention in older persons [Editorial]. *The Journals of Gerontology Series A: Biological Sciences and Medical Sciences, 57*, M338–M342.

Morrow-Howell, N. (2006–07). Civic service across the life course. *Generations, 30*, 37–42.

Morrow-Howell, N., & Freedman, M. (2006–07). Introduction: Bringing civic engagement into sharper focus. *Generations, 30*, 6–9.

Morrow-Howell, N., Hinterlong, J., Rozario, P. A., & Tang, F. (2003). Effects of volunteering on the well-being of older adults. *The Journals of Gerontology Series B: Psychological Sciences and Social Sciences, 58*, S137–S145.

Moxley, D. P., & Hyduk, C. A. (2003). The logic of personal advocacy with older adults and its implications for program management in community-based gerontology. *Administration in Social Work, 27*, 5–23.

Multicultural Mental Health Australia. (2003). Learning from experience: Community participation in the transcultural education of mental health professionals. *Synergy, 3*, 1–6.

Murphy, E. M. (2005). *Promoting healthy behavior.* Washington, DC: Population Reference Bureau.

Murphy, S., & Bennett, P. (2002). Psychology and health promotion. In R. Bunton & G. Macdonald (Eds.), *Health promotion: Disciplines, diversity and developments* (2nd ed., pp. 31–52). London: Routledge.

Myers, H. F., & Hwang, W. C. (2004). Cumulative psychosocial risks and resilience: A conceptual perspective on ethnic health disparities in late life. In N. B. Anderson, R. A. Bulatao, & B. Cohen (Eds.), *Critical perspectives on racial and ethnic differences in health in late life* (pp. 492–539). Washington, DC: National Academies Press.

Nadonezny, P. A., & Ojeda, M. (2005). Health services utilization between older and younger homeless adults. *Gerontologist, 45*, 249–254.

Naidoo, J., & Wills, J. (2000). *Health promotion: Foundation for practice* (2nd ed.). England: Bailliere Tindall.

Nakasato, Y. R., & Carnes, B. A. (2006). Health promotion in older adults. Promoting successful aging in primary care settings. *Geriatrics, 61*, 27–31.

Napoles-Springer, A. M., Santoyo, J., & Stewart, A. L. (2005). Recruiting ethnically diverse general internal medicine patients for a telephone survey on physician- patient communication. *Journal of General Internal Medicine, 20*, 438–443.

Narushima, M. (2004). A gaggle of raging grannies: The empowerment of older Canadian women through social activism. *International Journal of Lifelong Education, 23*, 23–42.

———. (2005). "Payback time": Community volunteering among older adults as a transformative mechanism. *Ageing & Society, 25*, 567–584.

Nash. C. (2001). The ageless self: Exploring holism. In A. Chiva & D. Stears (Eds.), *Promoting the health of older people* (pp. 63–70). Buckingham, England: Open University Press.

Nathonson, C. (1999). Social movements as catalysts for policy change: The case of tobacco control. *Journal of Health Politics Policy Law, 24*, 421–288.

National Association of Area Agencies on Aging. (2007). *Promoting the health, security and well-being of older adults: Policy priorities.* Washington, DC: Author.

National Association of Social Workers. (2003). *The aging of HIV.* Washington, DC: Author.

National Cancer Institute. (2007, July 27). Cancer prevention starts at home (with a party). *National Cancer Institute Bulletin, 4*, 1–2.

National Center for Health Statistics. (2006). National Nursing Home Survey (NNHS). Retrieved August 9, 2007, from the National Centers for Disease Control and Prevention website, www.cdc.gov/nchs/products/elecprods/subject/nnhs.htm.

National Center on Physical Activity and Disability. (2004). *Health promotion for people with disabilities: The amazing paradigm shift from disability prevention to prevention of secondary conditions.* Washington, DC: National Council on Aging.

National Diabetes Information Clearinghouse. (2005). *National estimates on diabetes.* Bethesda, MD: Author.

National Hispanic Council on Aging. (2005). *Improving the wellbeing of Latino older adults: Recommendations and solutions.* Washington, DC: Author.

National Institutes of Health. (2005, January 18). *Lifestyle changes especially effective at preventing type 2 diabetes in adults aged 60 and older.* Bethesda, MD: Author.

Nation's population one-third minority. (2006, May 10). *U.S. Census Bureau News.*

Neafsey, P. J. (2001). Adverse self-medication practices of older adults attending blood pressure clinics: Adverse self-medication practices. *Internet Journal of Advance Nursing Practice, 5.* Retrieved October 15, 2007, from www.ispub.com/ostia/index.php?xmlFilePath=journals/ijmh/vol1n1/self.xml.

Nelson-Lye, A. (2007, July 4). *Consumer models in health care. Do they really work?* Retrieved October 29, 2007, from www.nigeriavillagesquare.com.

Nestle, M., & Cowell, C. (1990). Health promotion for low-income minority groups: The challenge for nutrition education. *Health Education Research, 5*, 527–533.

Neundorfer, M. M., Camp, C. J., Lee, M. M., Skrajner, M. J., Malone, M. L., & Carr, J. R. (2004). Compensating for cognitive deficits in persons aged 50 and over with HIV/AIDS: A pilot study. In C. C. Poindexter & S. Keigher (Eds.), *Midlife and older adults and HIV: Implications for social service research, practice, and policy* (pp. 79–97). New York: Haworth Press.

New York State Office for the Aging. (2007). *Federal funding and policy priorities for the first session of the 110th Congress* (2007).

Newman, S., & Goff, R. (2006). Intergenerational relationships and civic engagement. In L. B. Wilson & S. P. Simson (Eds.), *Civic engagement and the baby boomer generation: Research, policy, and practice perspectives* (pp. 151–170). New York: Haworth Press.

News-Medical. Net. (2005, June 9). Healthy neighborhoods for older adults subject of study. Retrieved December 13, 2006, from www.news-medical.net?id=10856.

Nichols, J. E., Speer, D. C., Watson, B. J., Watson, M. R., Vergon, T. L., Vallee, C. M., et al. (2002). *Aging with HIV: Psychological, social, and health issues.* New York: Academic Press.

Nokes, K. M. (Ed.). (1996). *HIV/AIDS and the older adult.* Washington, DC: Taylor and Francis.

Nolan, J. (2001). Improving the health of older people: What do we do? *British Journal of Medicine, 10,* 524–528.

NOVA. (2004). *American Family: Aging in the Hispanic community.* Retrieved November 13, 2006, from www.pbs.org/americanfamily/aging.html.

Nutbeam, D., & Harris, E. (Eds.). (1999). *Theory in a nutshell: A guide to health promotion theory.* Sydney, Australia: McGraw-Hill.

O'Connell, J. J. (2005). *Premature mortality in homeless populations: A review of the literature.* Nashville, TN: National Health Care for the Homeless Council.

O'Connell, K. A. (2001). Smoking cessation among older clients. In E. A. Swanson, T. Tripp-Reimer, & K. Buckwalter (Eds.), *Health promotion and disease prevention in the older adult: Interventions and recommendations* (pp. 102–118). New York: Springer.

Odenheimer, G. L. (2006). Driver safety in older adults. The physician's role in assessing driving skills of older patients. *Geriatrics, 61,* 14–21.

Ohlemacher, S., & Callimachi, R. (2006, June 7). After hurricanes forced others away, Hispanics swept in. *Boston Globe,* p. A9.

Okoro, C. A., Young, S. L., Strine, T. W., Balluz, L. S., & Mokdad, A. H. (2004). Uninsured adults aged 65 years and older: Is their health at risk? *Journal of Health Care for the Poor and Underserved, 16,* 453–463.

Okun, M. A., & Michel, J. (2006). Sense of community and being a volunteer among the young-old. *Journal of Applied Gerontology, 25,* 173–188.

Oldenburg, B. R., Sallis, J. F., French, M. L., & Owen, N. (1999). Health promotion research and the diffusion and institutionalization of interventions. *Health Education Research, 14,* 121–130.

Older Women's Network. (2006a). *Aboriginal support circle.* Retrieved December 28, 2007, from www.own.org.au/aboriginalsupport.php.

———. (2006b). *About us: Guiding principles.* Retrieved November 14, 2007, from www.own.org.au/principles.php.

Oliver-Vazques, M., Sanchez-Ayendez, M., Suarez-Perez, E., Velez-Almodovar, H., & Arroyo-Calder, V. (2002). Breast cancer health promotion model for older Puerto Rican women: Results of a pilot programme. *Health Promotion International, 17,* 3–11.

O'Neill, G. (2005). *Civic engagement in an older America.* Washington, DC: The Gerontological Society of America.

———. (2006–07). Civic engagement on the agenda at the 2005 White House Conference on Aging. *Generations, 30,* 95–100.

O'Neill, P. (2002). *Caring for the older adult: A health promotion perspective.* Philadelphia, PA: Saunders.

Onge, J. S., Rogers, R., & Denney, J. (2004, August). *Obesity among black and white adults: The impact of place.* Paper presented at the annual meeting of the American Sociological Association, San Francisco.

Orel, N. A., Spence, M., & Steele, J. (2005). Getting the message out to older adults: Effective HIV health education risk reduction publications. *Journal of Applied Gerontology, 24*, 490–508.

Orel, N. A., Wright, J. M., & Wagner, J. (2004). Scarcity of HIV/AIDS risk-reduction materials targeting the needs of older adults among state departments of public health. *The Gerontologist, 44*, 693–696.

Orsega-Smith, E., Mowen, A. J., Payne, L. L., & Godbey, G. (2004). The interaction of stress and park use on psycho-physiological health in older adults. *Journal of Leisure Research, 36*, 232–256.

Ostir, G. V., Berges, I. M., Markides, K. S., & Ottenbacher, K. J. (2006). Hypertension in older adults and the role of positive emotions. *Psychosomatic Medicine, 68*, 727–733.

Ottawa Charter for Health Promotion. (1986). First International Conference on Health Promotion. Ottawa, WHO/HPR/HEP/95. 1.

Ozminkowski, R. J., Goetzel, R. Z., Wang, F., Gibson, T. B., Shechter, D., Musich, S., et al. (2006). The savings gained from participation in health promotion programs for Medicare beneficiaries. *Journal of Occupational and Environmental Medicine, 48*, 18.

Pandya, S. M. (2005). *Racial and ethnic differences among older adults in long-term care service use*. Washington, DC: AARP.

Pangman, V. C., & Seguire, M. (2000). Sexuality and the chronically ill older adult: A social justice issue. *Sexuality and Disability, 18*, 49–59.

Panter-Brick, C., Clarke, S. E., Lomas, H., Pinder, M., & Lindsey, S. W. (2006). Culturally compelling strategies for behaviour change: A social ecology model and case study on malaria prevention. *Social Science & Medicine, 62*, 2810–2825.

Patsdaughter, C. A., Christensen, M. H., Kelley, B. R., Masters, J. A., & Ndiwane, A. N. (2002). Meeting folks where they are: Collecting data from ethnic groups in the community. *Journal of Cultural Diversity, 9*, 26.

Pauline, J. S., Pauline, G. A., Johnson, S. R., & Gamble, K. M. (2006). Ethical issues in exercise psychology. *Ethics Behavior, 16*, 61–76.

Peale, I. (2004). Sexuality and sexual health promotion for the older person. *British Journal of Nursing, 13*, 188–193.

Pearsey, R. (2007, March 1). Racial healthcare gap persists. *UPI*. Retrieved August 16, 2007, from web.lexis-nexis.com/universe/document?_m=c468afe03b01054 f7394ea 79225df625.

Peck, M., & Hess, D. (2007, January 14). *Barriers to using public transit among diverse older adults: Implications for social work*. Retrieved September 21, 2007, from sswr .confex.com/sswr/2007/techprogram/P7047.HTM.

Peer Resources. (n.d.). The peer helping annotated and indexed bibliography. Retrieved June 18, 2007, from www.mentors.ca/Biblio5.html.

Penprase, B. (2006). Developing comprehensive health care for an underserved population. *Geriatric Nursing, 27*, 45–50.

Penson, R. T., Daniels, K. J., & Lynch, T. J. (2004). Too old to care? *Oncologist, 9*, 343–352.

Perkins, E. R., Simmett, J., & Wright, L. (Eds.). (1999a). Creative tensions in evidence-based practice. In E. R. Perkins, J. Simmett, J., & L. Wright. (Eds.), *Evidence-based health promotion* (pp. 1–21). New York: John Wiley & Sons.

Perkins, E. R., Simmett, J., & Wright, L. (Eds.). (1999b). *Evidence-based health promotion*. New York: John Wiley & Sons.

Perry, S. (2007, May 17). Baby boomers seek a purposeful direction in later life, study finds. *Chronicle of Philanthropy, 19*, 32.

Petry, N. M. (2002). A comparison of young, middle-aged, and older adult treatment-seeking pathological gamblers. *The Gerontologist, 42*, 92–99.

Petterson, J., Atwood, J. R., & Yates, B. (2002). Key elements for church-based health promotion programs: Outcome-based literature review. *Public Health Nursing, 19*, 401–411.

Pietrzak, R. H., Mollins, C. A., Ladd, G. T., Kerins, G. J., & Petry, N. M. (2005). Health and psychosocial correlates of disordered gambling in older adults. *American Journal of Geriatric Psychiatry, 13*, 510–519.

Pinn, J., Hill, S., Whitecross, P., Lloyd, B., & Pearce, C. (2006). *Kicking up autumn leaves: A report on the Women Owning Wellness Evaluation Project*. Sydney, Australia: OWN.

Poindexter, C. C. (2004). Six champions speak about being over 50 and living with HIV. In C. C. Poindexter & S. Keigher (Eds.), *Midlife and older adults and HIV: Implications for social service research, practice, and policy* (pp. 99–117). New York: Haworth Press.

Poindexter, C. C., & Emlet, C. (2006). HIV-infected and HIV-affected older adults. In B. Berkman & S. D'Ambruoso (Eds.), *Handbook of social work in health and aging* (pp. 91–99). New York: Oxford University Press.

Poindexter, C. C., & Krigher, S. M. (2004). Inclusion of "older" adults with HIV. In C. C. Poindexter & S. Keigher (Eds.), *Midlife and older adults and HIV: Implications for social service research, practice, and policy* (pp. 1–8). New York: Haworth Press.

Policy Research Associates. (2006). *Health care issues for older adults*. Delmar, NY: Author.

Polzer, R. L., & Miles, M. S. (2007). Spirituality in African Americans with diabetes: Self-management through relationship with God. *Qualitative Health Research, 17*, 176–188.

Popovic, J. R. (2001). *1999 National Hospital Discharge Survey: Annual summary with detailed diagnosis and procedure data*. National Center for Health Statistics Series Report 13(151), 154.

Population ageing: A looming public health challenge. (1998). *Health Millions, 24*, 20–22.

Potenza, M. N., Kosten, T. R., & Rounsaville, B. J. (2001). Pathological gambling. *Journal of the American Medical Society, 286*, 141–144.

PR Newswire. (2006a, November 14). Joslin's Latino Diabetes Initiative launches its first audio-novella for Hispanics/Latinos with diabetes and their families. Retrieved November 27, 2006, from www.highbeam.com/doc/1G1-154406156.html.

PR Newswire. (2006b, September 28). New report on caregiving warns "looming crisis" for baby boomers. Retrieved December 13, 2007, from www.schmiedingcenter.org.

Preston, F. W., Shapiro, P. D., & Keene, J. R. (2007). Successful aging and gambling: Predictors of gambling risk among older adults in Las Vegas. *American Behavioral Scientist, 51*, 102–121.

248 *Bibliography*

Prince. M., Patel, V., Saxena, S., Maselko, J., Phillips, M. R., & Rahman, A. (2007). No health without mental health. *The Lancet, 370,* 859–863.

Prison's ageing population: Over-60s are the fastest growing group of prisoners. (2006, September 7). *Community Care,* p. 30.

Pulloni, A. (2007). Health status of elderly Hispanics in the United States. In J. L. Angel & K. E. Whitfield (Eds.), *The health of aging Hispanics: The Mexican-origin population* (pp. 17–25). New York: Springer.

Purdie, N., & McCrindle, A. (2002). Self-regulation, self-efficacy and health behavior change in older adults. *Educational Gerontology, 28,* 379–400.

Pynoos, J., Rose, D., Rubenstein, L., Choi, I. H., & Sabata, D. (2006). Evidence-based interventions in fall prevention. *Home Health Care Services Quarterly, 25,* 55–73.

Quine, S., Kendig, H., Russell, C., & Touchard, D. (2004). Health promotion for socially disadvantaged groups: The case of homeless older men in Australia. *Health Promotion International, 19,* 157–165.

Quiroz-Martinez, J., Wu, D. P., & Zimmerman, K. (2005). *ReGeneration: Young people shaping environmental justice.* Oakland, CA: Movement Strategy Center.

Rabiner, D. J. (2005). Understanding the multidimensional nature of health promotion for older adults through the application of a conceptual framework. *Home Health Care Services Quarterly, 24,* 47–63.

Raeburn, J., & Corbett, T. (2001, May). *Community development: How effective is it an approach in health promotion?* Paper presented for the Second International Symposium on the Effectiveness of Health Promotion, University of Toronto.

Raphael, D. (2000). The question of evidence in health promotion. *Health Promotion International, 15,* 355–367.

Rawson, D. (2002). Health promotion theory and its rational reconstruction: Lessons from the philosophy of science. In R. Bunton & G. Macdonald (Eds.), *Health promotion: Disciplines, diversity and developments* (2nd ed., pp. 250–270). London: Routledge.

Raybould, C., & Adler, G. (2006). Applying NASW standards to end-of-life care for a culturally diverse aging population. *Journal of Social Work Values and Ethics, 3,* 2

Reilly, S. L. (2006). Transforming aging: The civic engagement of adults 55+. *Public Policy & Aging Report, 16,* 1, 3–8.

Resnick, B. (2000a). Health promotion practices of the older adult. *Public Health Nursing, 17,* 160–168.

———. (2000b). Hosting a wellness day: Promoting health in the old-old. *Clinical Excellence & Nursing Practice, 4,* 326–335.

———. (2001a). Geriatric health promotion. *Advanced Practice Nursing eJournal, 1.* Retrieved December 5, 2006, from www.medscape.com/viewarticle/408406_3.

———. (2001b). Promoting health in older adults: A four-year analysis. *Journal of the American Academy of Nursing Practice, 13,* 23–33.

———. (2003a). Health promotion practices of older adults: Model testing. *Public Health Nursing, 20,* 2–12.

———. (2003b). Health promotion practices of older adults: Testing and individualized approach. *Journal of Clinical Nursing, 12,* 46–55.

———. (2003c). Alcohol use in a continuing care retirement community. *Journal of Gerontological Nursing, 29,* 22–29.

Resnick, B., Vogel, A., & Luisi, D. (2006). Motivating minority older adults to exercise. *Cultural Diversity & Ethnic Minority Psychology, 12*, 17–29.

Resnick, D. B. (2007). Responsibility for health: Personal, social and environmental. *Journal of Medical Ethics, 33*, 444–445.

Rhea, M. K., Cook. C. B., El-Kebbi, I., Lyles, R. H., Dunbar, V. G., Panayloto, R. M., et al. (2005). Barriers to diabetes education in urban patients. *The Diabetes Educator, 31*, 410–417.

Rhodes, D. A., & Buchwald, D. (2003). Hypertension in older urban Native-American primary care patients. *Journal of the American Geriatrics Society, 51*, 774–781.

Richard, L., Gauvin, L., Ducharma, F., Gosselin, Sapinski, J. P., & Trudel, M. (2005). Health promotion and disease prevention for older adults: Intervention themes and strategies used in Quebec local community health centres and seniors' day centre. *Canadian Journal of Public Health, 96*, 467–470.

Richard, L., Laforest, S., Dufresne, F., & Sapinski, J. P. (2004). *The quality of life of older adults living in an urban environment: Professional and lay perspectives.* Toronto, Ontario, Canada: University of Toronto Press.

Richardson, J. (2002). Health promotion in palliative care: The patients' perception of therapeutic interaction with the palliative nurse in the primary care setting. *Journal of Advanced Nursing, 40*, 432–440.

Richardson, J. P. (2006, May 5). Considerations for health promotion and disease prevention in older adults. *Medscape Public Health & Prevention.* Retrieved September 25, 2006, from www.medscape.com/viewarticle/531942.

Rigaud, A. S., & Forette, B. (2001). Hypertension in older adults. *The Journals of Gerontology Series A: Biological Sciences & Medical Sciences, 56*, M217–M225.

Rimmer, J. H. (1999). Health promotion for people with disabilities: The emerging paradigm shift from disability prevention to prevention of secondary conditions, *Physical Therapy, 79*, 495–502.

Rissel, C. (1994). Empowerment: The holy grail of health promotion? *Health Promotion International, 9*, 39–47.

Roach III, M. (2000). Race and health: Implications for health care delivery and wellness promotion. In M. S. Jamner & D. Stokols (Eds.), *Promoting human wellness: New frontiers for research, practice, and policy* (pp. 258–293). Berkeley: University of California Press.

Robert Wood Johnson Foundation. (2007). *Findings brief: Meeting the future long-term care needs of the baby boomers.* Princeton, NJ: Author.

Robert, S. A., & Lee, K. Y. (2002). Explaining race differences in healthy older adults. *Research on Aging, 24*, 654–683.

Robinson, J. (2007, October 9). Competing and harmonizing in a Harlem pool. *New York Times*, p. C20.

Robinson, K. L., Driedger, M. S. Elliott, S. J., & Eyles, J. (2006). Understanding facilitators and barriers to health promotion practice. *Health Promotion Practice, 7*, 467–476.

Roff, L. L., Kiemmack, D. L., Parker, M., Koenig, H. G., Sawyer-Baker, P., & Altman, R. M. (2005). Religiosity, smoking, exercise, and obesity among Southern, community-dwelling older adults. *Journal of Applied Gerontology, 24*, 337–354.

Romero, S. M., Gerrard, M., & Owen, G. (2007). *Older adult civic engagement: A review of the non-profit sector's support systems and models.* St. Paul, MN: Saint Paul Foundation.

Rozario, P. A. (2006–07). Volunteering among current cohorts of older adults and baby boomers. *Generations, 30,* 31–36.

Rosen, L., Manor, O., Engelhard, D., & Zucker, D. (2006). In defense of the randomized controlled trial for health promotion research. *American Journal of Public Health, 96,* 1181–1186.

Rosenberg, E., & Letrero, I. L. (2006). Using age, cohort, and period to study elderly volunteerism. *Educational Gerontology, 32,* 313–334.

Roth, D. (2005). Culture change in long-term care: Educating the next generation. In H. R. moody (Ed.), *Religion, spirituality, and aging: A social work perspective* (pp. 233–248). New York: Haworth Press.

Roth, M. T., & Ivey, J. L. (2005). Self-reported medication use in community-residing older adults: A pilot study. *American Journal of Pharmacotherapy, 3,* 196–204.

Roubideaux, Y., Buchwald, D., Beals, J., Manson, S., Middlebrook, D., Muneta, B., et al. (2004). Measuring the quality of diabetes care for older American Indians and Alaska Natives. *American Journal of Public Health, 94,* 60–65.

Ruffing-Rahal, M. A. (1991). Rationale and design for health promotion with older adults. *Public Health Nursing, 8,* 258–263.

Sadler, G. R., York, C., Madlensky, L., Gibson, K., Wasserman, L., Rosenthal, E., et al. (2006). Health parties for African American study recruitment. *Journal of Cancer Education, 21,* 71–76.

Sahay, T. S., Ashbury, F. D., Roberts, M., & Rootman, I. (2006). Effective components for nutrition interventions: A review and application of the literature. *Health Promotion Practice, 7,* 418–427.

Saint Paul Foundation. (2007). *The civic engagement of baby boomers: Preparing for a new wave of volunteers.* St. Paul, MN: Author.

Sambamoorthi, U., & Findley, P. (2004). Who are the elderly who never receive influenza immunization? *Preventive Medicine, 40,* 469–478.

Sandefur, G. D., Campbell, M. E., & Eggerling-Boeck. J. (2004). Racial and ethnic identification, official classifications, and health disparities. In N. B. Anderson, R. A. Bulatao, & B. Cohen (Eds.), *Critical perspectives on racial and ethnic differences in health in late life* (pp. 25–52). Washington, DC: National Academies Press.

Sander, T. H., & Putnam, R. D. (2006). Social capital and civic engagement of individuals over age fifty in the United States. In L. B. Wilson & S. P. Simson (Eds.), *Civic engagement and the baby boomer generation: Research, policy, and practice perspectives* (pp. 21–39). New York: Haworth Press.

Sands, D. R. (2005, November 24). Europe's "baby bust" signals major change; military, economic strength may falter. *Washington Times,* p. A01.

Santos-Ortiz, M. del C., Matte, H., Correa-Nivar, K., & Pintado-Diaz, E. (2004). HIV/ AIDS among middle and older adults in Puerto Rico. *California Journal of Health Promotion, 2,* 30–39.

Saskatchewan Health. (2003). *Evidence supporting population health promotion initiatives.* Regina, Saskatchewan, Canada: Population Health Branch.

Satre, D. D., & Arean, P. A. (2005). Effects of gender, ethnicity, and medical illness on drinking cessation in older primary care patients. *Journal of Aging and Health, 17,* 70–84.

Scandlyn, J. (2000). When AIDS became a chronic disease. *Western Journal of Medicine, 172,* 130–133.

Schensul, J. J., Disch, W. B., Vazquez, E., Radda, K. E., & Jepsen, R. (2006). *Pilot results from a flu vaccine uptake empowerment intervention with older minority and low income adults.* Paper presented at the 2006 National Immunization Conference.

Schibusawa, T. (2006). Older adults with substance/alcohol abuse problems. In B. Berkman & S. D'Ambruoso (Eds.), *Handbook of social work in health and aging* (pp. 141–147). New York: Oxford University Press.

Schiller, J. S., & Ni, H. (2006). Cigarette smoking and smoking cessation among persons with chronic obstructive pulmonary disease. *American Journal of Health Promotion, 20,* 319–323.

Schneider, E. C., Altpeter, M., & Whitelaw, N. (2007). An innovative approach for building health promotion program capacity: A generic volunteer training curriculum. *The Gerontologist, 47,* 398–403.

Schoeni, R. F., Freedman, V. A., & Martin, L. G. (2005). *Socioeconomic and demographic disabilities in trends in old-age disability.* Ann Arbor, MI: Institute for Social Research, University of Michigan.

Schrimshaw, E. W. (2003). Perceived barriers to social support from families and friends among older adults with HIV/AIDS. *Journal of Health Psychology, 8,* 738–752.

Schroeder, P. (2007, June 10). *Principles for public health ethics: A practical framework for ethical challenges in population wide health promotion.* Bielefeld, Germany: Institute of Public Health NRW.

Schuler, P. B., Roy, J. L. P., Vinci, D., Philipp, S. F., & Cohen, S. J. (2006). Barriers and motivations to exercise in older African American and European American women. *California Journal of Health Promotion, 4,* 128–134.

Schulz, A., & Northridge, M. E. (2004). Social determinants of health: Implications for environmental health promotion. *Health Education & Behavior, 31,* 455–471.

Schwartz, C., Meisenhelder, J. B., Ma, Y., & Reed, G. (2003). Altruistic social interest behaviors are associated with better mental health. *Psychosomatic Medicine, 65,* 778–785.

Seeman, T. E. (2000). Health promoting effects of friends and family on health outcomes in older adults. *American Journal of Health Promotion, 14,* 362–370.

Shah, M. N., Bazarian, J. J., Lerner, E. B., Fairbanks, R. J., Barker, W. H., Auinger, P., et al. (2007). The epidemiology of emergency medical services by older adults: An analysis of the National Hospital Ambulatory Medical Care Survey. *Academy of Emergency Medicine, 14,* 441–447.

Shankle, M. D., Maxwell, C. A., Katzman, E. S., & Landers, S. (2003). An invisible population: Older lesbian, gay, bisexual, and transgender individuals. *Clinical Research and Regulatory Affairs, 20,* 159–182.

Shaping the future of health promotion: Priorities for action. (2008). *Health Promotion International, 23,* 98–102.

Sheth, A. N., Moore, R. D., & Gebo, K. A. (2006). Provision of general and HIV-specific health maintenance in middle aged and older patients in an urban HIV clinic. *AIDS Patient Care & STDS, 20,* 318–325.

Shippy, R. A., & Karpiak, S. E. (2005). Perceptions of support among older adults with HIV. *Research on Aging, 27,* 290–306.

Showkeir, J. R. (1974). Tapping "older" energy resources: One of many undiscovered—unused community assets. *Community Education Journal, 4,* 46–48.

Silva, P., & Thomas, C. (2006). Civic engagement and national service: Results from Senior Corps evaluations. In L. B. Wilson & S. P. Simson (Eds.), *Civic engagement and the baby boomer generation: Research, policy, and practice perspectives* (pp. 43–60). New York: Haworth Press.

Simpson, C. (2004). When hope makes us vulnerable: A discussion of patient–healthcare provider interactions in the context of hope. *Bioethics, 18,* 428–447.

Sindall, C. (2002). Does health promotion need a code of ethics? *Health Promotion International, 17,* 201–203.

Singal, A. (2006, November 7). The diet connection for Hispanics. Dallas Morning News.Com. Retrieved November 6, 2007, from www.dallasnews.com/shared-content/dws/fea/taste/easyrecipes/stories/DN-NH_hispa.

Sirianni. C., & Friedland, L. (2001). *Civic innovation in America: Community empowerment, public policy, and the movement for civic renewal.* Berkeley: University of California Press.

Smith, M. W., Levy, J. A., & Schensul, J. (2002). *Older minority adult attitudes toward AIDS and people with AIDS.* International Conference on AIDS, July 7–12, Abstract No. E11703.

Song, J., Chang, H. J., Tirodkar, M., Cheng, R. W., Manheim, L. M., & Dunlop, D. D. (2007). Racial/ethnic differences in activities of daily living disability in older adults with arthritis: A longitudinal study. *Arthritis Care & Research, 57,* 1058–1066.

Sotomayor, M., Pawlik, F., & Dominguez, A. (2007). Building community capacity for health promotion in a Hispanic community. *Prevention of Chronic Diseases, 4,* A16.

Squire, A. (2001). Health-promoting residential settings. In A. Chiva & D. Stears (Eds.), *Promoting the health of older people* (pp. 120–131). Buckingham, England. Open University Press.

States, R. A., Susman, W. M., Riquelme, L. F., Goodwin, E. M., & Greer, E. (2006). Community health education: Reaching ethnically diverse elders. *Journal of Allied Health, 35,* 215–222.

Staudinger, U. M., Kessier, E. M., & Dorner, J. (2006). Wisdom in social context. In K. Warner Schaie & L. L. Carstensen (Eds.), *Social structures, aging, and self-regulation in the elderly* (pp. 33–53). New York: Springer.

Sterman, J. D. (2006). Learning from evidence in a complex world. *American Journal of Public Health, 96,* 505–514.

Sternberg, Z., Munschauer III, F. E., Carrow, S. S., & Sternberg, E. (2006). Faith-placed cardiovascular health promotion: A framework for contextual and organizational factors underlying program success. *Health Education Research, 22,* 619–629.

Stevens, J. A. (2006, November 17). Fatalities and injuries from falls among older adults United States, 1993–2003 and 2001–2005. *Morbidity and Mortality Weekly Report, 55,* 1221–1224.

Stevens, J. A., & Olson, S. (2000). Reducing falls and resulting hip fractures among older women. In CDC recommendations regarding selected conditions affecting women's health. *MMWR, 49*(RR–2), 3–12.

Stevens, J. A., Corso, P. S., Finkelstein, E. A., & Miller, T. R. (2006). The costs of fatal and nonfatal falls among older adults. *Injury Prevention, 12*, 290–295.

Stevens, J. A., Hasbrouck, L. M., Durant, T. M., Dellinger, A. M., Batabyal, P. K., Crosby, A. E., et al. (1999, December 17). Surveillance for injuries and violence among older adults. *MMWR, 48*(SS08), 27–50.

Stewart, A. L., Gillis, D., Grossman, M., Castrillo, M., Pruitt, L., McLellan, B., et al. (2006). Diffusing a research-based physical activity promotion program for seniors into diverse communities: CHAMPS III. *Preventing Chronic Disease* [online]. Retrieved July 2, 2007 from www.cdc.gov/pcd/issues/2006/ apr/05_0091.htm.

Stokols, D. (2000). The social ecological paradigm of wellness promotion. In M. S. Jamner & D. Stokols (Eds.), *Promoting human wellness: New frontiers for research, practice, and policy* (pp. 21–37). Berkeley: University of California Press.

Stone, L. C., Viruell-Fuentes, E. A., & Acevedo-Garcia, D. (2007). Understanding the socio-economic, health systems & policy threats to Latino health: Gaining new perspectives for the future. *California Journal of Health Promotion, 5*, 82–104.

Story, L. (2007). Principles of community social change and empowerment supporting health promotion. *Helium Society & Lifestyles.* Retrieved November 19, 2007, from www.helium.com/tm/145283/principles-empowerment-social-changewallerstein.

Struck, B. D., & Ross, K. M. (2006). Health promotion in older adults: Prescribing exercise for the frail and home bound. *Geriatrics, 61*, 22–27.

Substance Abuse and Mental Health Services Administration. (2002). *Substance use by older adults: Estimates of future impact on the treatment system.* Rockville, MD: Author.

———. (2006a, May 5). Older adults in substance abuse treatment: Update. *The DASIS Report*, 1–5.

———. (2006b). *Substance abuse among older adults: 2002 and 2003 update.* Washington, DC: Author.

Sudore, R. L., Yaffe, K., Satterfield, S., Harris, T. B., Mehta, K. M., Simonsick, E. M., et al. (2006). Limited literacy and mortality in the elderly: The health, aging, and body composition study. *Journal of General Internal Medicine, 21*, 806–812.

Sullivan, K., Lynch, A., Artesani, A., & Seed, S. (2007). Medicine and alcohol misuse among older adults. *U.S. Pharmacy, 32*, HS20–HS30.

Sullivan, W. C., Kuo, F. E., & Depooter, S. F. (2004). The fruit of urban nature. *Environment and Behavior, 36*, 678–700.

Surbone, A., Kagawa-Singer, M., Teret, C., & Baider, L. (2006). The illness trajectory of elderly cancer patients across cultures: SIOG position paper. *Annals of Oncology, 18*, 633–638.

Sutherland, M., Cowar, M., & Heck, C. (1988). A community organization: Peer facilitated senior citizen health promotion program. *International Quarterly of Community Health Education, 8*, 181–187.

Sutton, S. E., & Kemp, S. P. (2006). Integrating social science and design inquiry through interdisciplinary design charrettes: *An approach to participatory community problem solving. American Journal of Community Psychology, 38*, 125–139.

Swerissen, H., & Crisp, B. R. (2004). The sustainability of health promotion interventions for different levels of social organization. *Health Promotion International, 19,* 123–130.

Syme, S. L. (2000). Community participation, empowerment, and health: Development of a wellness guide for California. In M. S. Jamner & D. Stokols (Eds.), *Promoting human wellness: New frontiers for research, practice, and policy* (pp. 78–98). Berkeley: University of California Press.

Szczepura, A. (2006). Access to health care for ethnic minority populations. *Postgraduate Medical Journal, 81,* 141–147.

Szerlip, M. A., DeSalvo, K. B., & Szerlip, H. M. (2005). Predictors of HIV-infection in older adults. *Journal of Aging Health, 17,* 293–304.

Tagliareni, M. E., & King, E. S. (2006). Documenting health promotion services in community-based nursing centers, *Holistic Nursing Practice, 20,* 20–26.

Tan, E. J., Xue, Q., Li, T., Carlson, M. C., & Fried, L. P. (2006). Volunteering: A physical activity intervention for older adults: The Experience Corps program in Baltimore. *Journal of Urban Health: Bulletin of the New York Academy of Medicine.* (www.jhsph.edu/agingandhealth). Accessed June 17, 2007.

Tannahill, A. (1985). What is health promotion? *Health Promotion Journal, 44,* 167–168.

Tatara, T. (Ed.). (1999). *Understanding elder abuse in minority populations.* Phildalephia, PA: Brunner/Mazel.

Texas Cooperative Extension. (2006). *Minority Peer Educator Project.* College Station: Texas A&M University, Family and Consumer Sciences.

Texas Department on Aging. (2003). *Texas demographics: Older adults in Texas.* Austin: Author.

Thoits, P. A., & Hewitt, L. N. (2001). Volunteer work and well-being. *Journal of Health and Social Behavior, 42,* 115–131.

Thorogood, M. (2002). What is the relevance of sociology for health promotion? In R. Bunton & G. Macdonald (Eds.), *Health promotion: Disciplines, diversity and developments* (2nd ed., pp. 53–79). London: Routledge.

Thorogood, M., & Coombes, Y. (Eds.). (2004). *Evaluating health promotion practice and methods.* New York: Oxford University Press.

Tilford, S. (2000). Evidence-based health promotion. *Health Education Research, 15,* 659–663.

Tjia, J., Givens, J. L., Karlawish, J. H., Okoli-Umeweni, A., & Barg, F. K. (2007). Beneath the surface: Discovering the unvoiced concerns of older adults with type 2 diabetes mellitus. *Health Education Research, 23,* 40–52.

Tomes, N. (2006). The patient as a policy factor: A historical case study of the consumer/ survivor movement in mental health. *Health Affairs, 25,* 720–729.

Tomita, S. (2006). Mistreated and neglected elders. In B. Berkman & S. D'Ambruoso (Eds.), *Handbook of social work in health and aging* (pp. 219–230). New York: Oxford University Press.

Torres, I. (2004). *Rethinking the demographics of addiction: Helping older adults find recovery.* Rockville, MD: Substance Abuse and Mental Health Services Administration.

Transportation Research Board. (2004). *Transportation in an aging society: A decade of experience.* Washington, DC: Author.

Trevino, F., & Coustasse, A. (2007). Disparities and access barriers to health care among Mexican American elders. In J. L. Angel & K. E. Whitfield (Eds.), *The health of aging Hispanics: The Mexican-origin population* (pp. 165–180). New York: Springer.

Trinitapoli, J. (2005). Congregation-based services for elders. *Research on Aging, 27,* 241–264.

Tudor-Locke, C., Henderson, K. A., Wilcox, S., Cooper, R. S. Durstine, J. L., & Ainsworth, B. E. (2003). In their own voice: Definitions and interpretations of physical activity. *Women's Health Issues, 13,* 194–199.

Tummers, N., & Hendrick, F. (2007, March). Older adults say yes to yoga. *National Recreation and Park Administration,* pp. 1–3.

Tuokko, H. A., Rhodes, R. E & Dean, R. (2007). Health conditions, heart symptoms and driving difficulties in older adults. *Age and Ageing, 36,* 389–394.

Tzoulas, K., Korpeta, K. Venn, S., Yli-Pelkonen, V., Kazmierczak, A., Niemela, J., et al. (2007). Promoting ecosystem and human health in urban areas using green infrastructure: A literature review. *Landscape and Urban Planning, 81,* 167–178.

U.S. Administration on Aging. (2006). Health promotion and disease prevention for older adults: Programs that work. *Prevention Report, 20,* 1–6.

U.S. Census Bureau. (2007). *Older adults in 2005.* Washington, DC: Author.

Valcour, V., & Paul, R. (2006). HIV infection and demenitia in older adults. *Clinical Infectious Diseases, 42,* 1449–1454.

Valente, T. W. (2002). *Evaluating health promotion programs.* New York: Oxford University Press.

Valle, R., Yamada, A. M., & Matiella, A. C. (2006). Fotonovelas: A health literacy tool for educating Latino older adults about dementia. *Clinical Gerontologist, 30,* 71–88.

Van Willigen, M. (2000). Differential benefits of volunteering across the life course. *The Journals of Gerontology Series B: Psychological Sciences and Social Sciences, 55,* S308–S318.

Vance, D. E., & Robinson, F. P. (2004). Reconciling successful aging with HIV: A bio-psychosocial overview. In C. C. Poindexter & S. Keigher (Eds.), *Midlife and older adults and HIV: Implications for social service research, practice, and policy* (pp. 59–78). New York: Haworth Press.

Vann, K. (2006, September 13). It's an age-old story, unfortunately; elderly taught how to fight age discrimination. *Hartford Courant* (Connecticut), p. D1.

Vasquez, V. B., Lanza, D., Hennessey-Lavery, S., Fascente, S., Halpin, H. A., & Minkler, M. (2007). Addressing food security through public policy action in a community-based participatory research partnership. *Health Promotion Practice, 8,* 342–349.

Vickers, K. (2007). Aging and the media: Yesterday, today, and tomorrow. *California Journal of Health Promotion, 3,* 100–105.

Vlahov, D., Freudenberg, N., Proietti, F., Quinn, D., Nadi, V., & Galea, S. (2007). Urban as a determinant of health. *Journal of Urban health, 84*(Suppl 1), 16–26.

Vlahov, D., & Galea, S. (2002). Urbanization, urbanicity, and health. *Journal of Urban Health, 79*(Suppl 4), S1–S12.

Volland, P. J., & Berkman, B. (2004). Educating social workers to meet the challenge of an aging urban population: A promising model. *Academy of Medicine, 79,* 1192–1197.

Wakefield, S., Yeudall, F., Taron, C., Reynolds, J., & Skinner, A. (2007). Growing urban health: Community gardening in South-East Toronto. *Health Promotion International, 22*, 92–101.

Walker, J. (2001). Health and productive aging. In A. Chiva & D. Stears (Eds.), *Promoting the health of older people* (pp. 73–85). Buckingham, England: Open University Press.

Wallace, L. S. (2004). The impact of limited literacy on health promotion in the elderly. *California Journal of Health Promotion, 2*, 1–4.

Wallerstein. N., & Freudenberg, N. (1998). Linking health promotion and social justice: A rationale and two case studies. *Health Education Research, 13*, 451–457.

Warren-Findlow, J., Prohaska, T. R., & Freedman, D. (2003). Challenges and opportunities in recruiting and retaining underrepresented populations into health promotion research. *The Gerontologist, 43*, 37–46.

Washington, O. G. (2005). Identification and characteristics of older homeless African American women. *Issues in Mental Health Nursing, 26*, 117–136.

Waters, C. M. (2001). Understanding and supporting African Americans' perspectives of end-of-life care planning and decision making. *Qualitative Health Research, 11*, 385–398.

Waters, C. M. (2000). End-of-life directives among African Americans: Lessons learned—a need for community-centered discussion and education. *Journal of Community Health Nursing, 17*, 25–37.

Weed, D. L., & McKeown, R. E. (2003). Science, ethics, and professional public health practice. *Journal of Epidemiology and Community Health, 57*, 4–5.

Weinrich, S. P., Weinrich, M. C., Stromborg, M. F., Boyd, M. D., & Weiss, H. L. (1993). Using elderly educators to increase coloerectal cancer screening. *The Gerontologist, 33*, 491–496.

Weiss, S. C., & Gomperts, J. S. (2005). The value of experience. *Educational Leadership, 62*, 22–27.

Weitzman, P. F., & Levkoff, S. E. (2000). Combining qualitative and quantitative methods in health research with minority elders: Lessons from a study of dementia caregiving. *Field Methods, 12*, 195–208.

Wenzel, E. (1997). A comment on settings in health promotion. *Internet Journal of Health Promotion.* Retrieved August 7, 2006, from www.ldb.org/setting.htm.

Whelan, R. (2007, October 8). China's age-old problem. *The Irish Times, 54.*

White, M. C., Tulsky, J. P., Dawson, C., Zolopa, A. R., & Moss, A. R. (1997). Association between time homeless and perceived health status among the homeless in San Francisco. *Journal of Community Health, 22*, 271–282.

Whitehead, D. (2006). The health promoting prison (HPP) and its imperative for nursing. *International Journal of Nursing Studies, 43*, 123–131.

Whitehead, S., Baxendale, A., Bryee, C., MacHardy, L., Young, I., & Witney, E. (2001). "Settings" based health promotion: A review. *Health Promotion International, 16*, 339–353.

Whitfield, K. E., & Hayward, M. (2003). The landscape of health disparities among older adults. *Public Policy & Aging Report, 13*, 1–22.

Wilbur, J., McDevitt, J., Wang, E., Dancy, B., Briller, J., Ingram, D., et al. (2006). Recruitment of African American women to a walking program: Eligibility, ineligibility, and attrition during screening, *Researching Nursing Health, 29,* 176–189.

Wieck, K. L. (2000). Health promotion for inner-city minority elderly. *Journal of Community Health Nursing, 17,* 131–139.

Wieringa, M. H., Vermeire, P. A., Bever, H. P. V., Nelen, V. J., & Weyler, J. J. (2001). Higher occurrence of asthma-related symptoms in an urban than a suburban area in adults, but not in children. *European Respiratory Journal, 17,* 422–427.

Wight, R. G., Aneshensel, C. S., Miller-Martinez, D., Botticello, A. L., Cummings, J. R., Karlamangla, A. S., et al. (2006). Urban neighborhood context, educational attainment, and cognitive function among older adults. *American Journal of Epidemiology, 163,* 1071–1078.

Wilcox, S., Laken, M., Anderson, T., Bopp, M., Bryant, D., Cater, R., et al. (2007). The Health-e-AME Faith-Based Physical Activity Initiative: Description and baseline findings. *Health Promotion Practice, 8,* 69–78.

Wilken, C. S. (2002). *Myths and realities of aging.* Gainsville: University of Florida IFAS Extension.

Wilken, C. S., & Walker, K. (2003). *Ethical issues in building and maintaining coalitions: A 10-step decision-making model for choosing between right and right.* Gainsville: University of Florida, IFAS Extension.

Wilkins, C. H., Wilkins, K. L., Meisel, M., Depke, M. S., Williams, J., & Edwards, D. F. (2007). Dementia undiagnosed in poor older adults with functional impairments. *Journal of the Ameican Geriatrics Society, 55,* 1771–1776.

Willard, S., & Dean, L. M. (2000). AIDS in the elderly. Aging raises unique treatment concerns. *Advance Nursing Practice, 8,* 54–58.

Williams, E., & Donnelly, J. (2002). Older Americans and AIDS: Some guidelines for prevention. *Social Work, 47,* 105–111.

Wilmoth, J. M., & Longino, C. F. (2006). Demographic trends that will shape U.S. policy in the twenty-first century. *Research on Aging, 28,* 269–288.

Wilson, L. B., & Rymph, D. B. (2006). Research issues in civic engagement: Outcomes of a national agenda-setting meeting. In L. B. Wilson & S. P. Simson (Eds.), *Civic engagement and the baby boomer generation: Research, policy, and practice perspectives* (pp. 195–211). New York: Haworth Press.

Wilson, L. B., & Simson, S. P. (Eds.). (2006a). *Civic engagement and the baby boomer generation: Research, policy, and practice perspectives.* New York: Haworth Press.

Wilson, L. B., & Simson, S. P. (2006b). Civic engagement research, policy, and practice priority areas: Future perspectives on the baby boomer generation. In L. B. Wilson & S. P. Simson (Eds.), *Civic engagement and the baby boomer generation: Research, policy, and practice perspectives* (pp. 247–265). New York: Haworth Press.

Wilson, L. B., Steele, J., Simson, S. P., & Harlow-Rosentraub, K. (2006). Legacy Leadership Institutes: Combining lifelong learning with civic engagement. In L. B. Wilson & S. P. Simson (Eds.), *Civic engagement and the baby boomer generation: Research, policy, and practice perspectives* (pp. 111–141). New York: Haworth Press.

Wilson, N., Desho, S., Martin, A. C., Wallerstein, N., Wang, C. C., & Minkler, M. (2007). Engaging young adolescents in social action through photovoice. *The Journal of Early Adolescence, 27,* 241–261.

Windsor, T. D., & Anstey, K. J. (2006). Interventions to reduce the adverse psychosocial impact of driving cessation on older adults. *Clinical Interventions in Aging, 1,* 205–211.

Winningham, A., Corwin, S., Moore, C., Richter, D., Sargent, R., & Gore-Felton, C. (2004). The changing age of HIV: Sexual risk among older African American women living in rural communities. *Preventive Medicine, 39,* 809–814.

Winningham, A., Richter, D., Corwin, S., & Gore-Felton, C. (2004). Perceptions of vulnerability to HIV among older African American women: The role of intimate partners. In C. C. Poindexter & S. Keigher (Eds.), *Midlife and older adults and HIV: Implications for social service research, practice, and policy* (pp. 25–42). New York: Haworth Press.

Wolf, M. S., Gazmararian, J. A., & Baker, D. W. (2005). Health literacy and functional health status among older adults. *Archives of Internal Medicine, 165,* 1946–1952.

Wolf, S. L., O'Grady, M., Easley, K. A., Guo, Y., Kressig, R. W., & Kutner, M. (2006). The influence of intense Tai Chi training on physical performance and hemo-dynamic outcomes in transitionally frail, older adults. *The Journals of Gerontology Series A: Biological Sciences & Medical Sciences, 61,* 184–189.

Wycherley, B. (2001). Lifeskills: From adaptation to transcendence. In A. Chiva & D. Stears (Eds.), *Promoting the health of older people* (pp. 51–62). Buckingham, England: Open University Press.

Wygant. S. (2007, August 21). Diagnosis: Alzheimer's disease; risk factors & treatment options. *News and Commentary on Issues Impacting Seniors in Michigan.* Retrieved October 20, 2007, from http://homeinstead.wordpress.com/2007/08/21/diagnosis-alzheimers-disease-risk-factors-tr.

Wyman, J. F. (2001). Exercise interventions. In E. A. Swanson, T. Tripp-Reimer, & K. Buckwalter (Eds.), *Health promotion and disease prevention in the older adult: Interventions and recommendations* (pp. 1–42). New York: Springer.

Yamada, A. M., Valle, R., Barrio, C., & Jeste, D. (2006). Selecting an acculturation measure with Latino older adults. *Research on Aging, 28,* 519–561.

Yanek, L. R., Becker, D. M., Moy, T. F., Gittelsohn, J., & Koffman, D. M. (2001). Project Joy: Faith-based cardiovascular health promotion for African American women. *Public Health Report, 116,* 68–81.

Yee, B. W. K., & Weaver, G. D. (1994). Ethnic minorities and health promotion: Developing a "culturally competent" agenda. *Generation, 18,* 39–44.

Yeh, M. C., Ickes, S. B., Lowenstein, L. M., Shuval, K., Ammerman, A. S., Farris, R., et al. (2008). Understanding barriers and facilitators of fruit and vegetable consumption among a diverse multi-ethnic population in the USA. *Health Promotion International, 23,* 42–51.

Yorston, G. A., & Taylor, P. J. (2006). Commentary: Older offenders—No place to go? *Journal of the American Academy of Psychiatry & Law, 34,* 333–337.

Young, A. S., Chinman, M., Forquer, S. L., Knight, E. L., Vogel, H., Miller, A., et al. (2005). Use of consumer-led intervention to improve provider competencies. *Psychiatric Services, 56,* 967–975.

Young, L. E., & Hayes, V. E. (Eds.). (2002). *Transforming health promotion practice: concepts, issues, and applications.* Philadelphia, PA: F. A. Davis Company.

Young, R. F. (1993). Health promotion among minority aged: Challenges for the health professions. *Journal of Continuing Education in the Health Professions, 13,* 235–242.

Zaranek, R. R., & Chapleski, E. F. (2005). Casino gambling among urban elders: Just another social activity? *Journals of Gerontology B, 60,* S74–S81.

Zedlewski, S. R., & Schaner, S. G. (2006). Older adults engaged as volunteers. *Perspectives on Productive Aging, 5,* 1–7.

Zenk, S. N., Schulz, A. J., Israel, B. A., James, D., Bao, S., & Wilson, M. L. (2005). Neighborhood racial composition, neighborhood poverty, and spatial accessibility of supermarkers in metropolitan Detroit. *American Journal of Public Health, 95,* 660–667.

Zodikoff, B. D. (2006). Services for lesbian, gay, bisexual, and transgendered older adults. In B. Berkman & S. D'Ambruoso (Eds.), *Handbook of social work in health and aging* (pp. 569–575). New York: Oxford University Press.

Index

Index